HOMOEOPATHY FOR
ILLNE

By the same author:-

Homoeopathic Medicine

The Homoeopathic Treatment of Emotional Illness

A Woman's Guide to Homoeopathy

Understanding Homoeopathy

Talking About Homoeopathy

An Encyclopedia of Homoeopathy

The Principles, Art and Practice of Homoeopathy

Emotional Health

Personal Growth and Creativity

The Side-Effects Book

Homoeopathy for Pregnancy and Nursing Mothers

Homoeopathy for Babies and Children

Homoeopathy for Everyday Stress Problems

Homoeopathy for Teenager Problems

Homoeopathy for the Menopause

HOMOEOPATHY FOR PSYCHOLOGICAL ILLNESS

A Guide to Mental Health Problems

by

Dr Trevor Smith
MA, MB, BChir, DPM, MFHom

INSIGHT

Insight Editions
Worthing, Sussex
England

WARNING

The contents of this volume are for general interest only and individual persons should always consult their medical adviser about a particular problem or before stopping or changing an existing treatment.

Published by Insight Editions 1994
Worthing
Sussex
England

© Trevor Smith 1994

Trevor Smith asserts the moral right to
be identified as the author of this work.

British Library Cataloguing in Publication Data

**A catalogue record for this book is available
from the British Library.**

ISBN 0-496670 20 X

Cover photograph by the author.

INTRODUCTION

In health, we are aware of having a personal inner self, which thinks and feels. Also that there are others, outside of us, who are quite separate and different.

The totality of our inner thoughts, feelings, and memories, we call mind. We may choose or not, to communicate it to others, depending on the closeness of the individual relationship and the degree of trust which exists.

What 'you' or others say, the external signals 'I' receive, process and react to all the time, are outside the essential 'me' and something other than my personal individuality and identity.

In health, there is a clear-cut distinct boundary between what is self (or 'me'), and what is 'you' (or other). A clear difference exists between what I think, say and want, and what you say, think, or demand.

I know what is 'me', what I want, feel and think, but I can only guess what 'you' are thinking. I can never get inside your mind and know you as well as I know myself.

The combinations of different ways of thinking, feeling, needs and reactions in changing different situations, makes up our personality. These inner needs and feelings, their depth, strength and intensity, are our sense of identity which give it character and confidence.

The mind interprets and co-ordinates, makes sense of a wide variety of reactions and signals (flashes of energy), from many different internal areas:- emotional reactions, instincts, conditioned responses, thoughts, experience, intuitive feelings and memories. Together with input from outside external sources, particularly visual and auditory impressions, they create a recognizable pattern and framework, we can understand and respond to.

The mind is situated within the brain and depends upon it for healthy functioning.

If the brain is physically ill, drugged, or senile, the mind is also affected, as can be clearly seen in a child or adult with a high fever, or when coming round from a general anaesthetic. At such times, disorientated, confused and overactive patterns of behaviour may occur with misperception of others, and events around us. Senile dementia may lead to hallucinations, violence, or delusional (distorted and unreal) thinking. There may be a conviction that the family is 'telling lies' i.e. trying to get rid of them, stealing personal items, or in some way plotting against them.

In an extreme pressure situation, as occurs when under severe stress, all the feelings become pressurised and intensified with a surge of restless excitement, extremes of emotion and irritability. If this continues to build-up, there is a risk of loss of control and eventually an emotional breakdown with a flood of emotions which cannot be held in check.

With too much accumulated emotion, the thought processes may become fragmented. Thoughts are shed or detached from the mind, only to return and bombard it with need, demand, and compulsive feelings. The conviction that someone external must have placed the fragmented thoughts inside the mind, leads to an impression of being under the control of others, heightening anxiety, fear, mistrust and aggression. Loss of confidence occurs. As suspicion and mistrust build-up, this may further heighten internal tensions, adding to pressures which fragment coherent (logical) thoughts and ideas.

Thinking may eventually become totally distorted, with a dissociated spaced-out sensation, lacking concentration, difficulty in focusing attention, and eventually leading to confusion and the breakdown of organised thinking. Paranoid (or persecutory) feelings, reflect hostile, resentful, negative attitudes towards others, with feelings of suspicion and often inappropriate behaviour. Others are felt to be plotting, and seeking to undermine position and security.

A paranoid persecutory illness may develop, as emotions become fragmented in the same way as the thought processes. All the internal processes of the mind may seem to be scattered, leading to a sense of non-existence, delusions of being already 'dead', part of the galaxy, or floating in space. At times there may be a feeling of being in a vacuum or sucked out like a shell, perhaps turned into a radio speaker, transparent and vulnerable. The inside of the body may feel made of glass and about to shatter at any moment. At other times there is a feeling of God-like omnipotence, of power or peace, and able to embrace the universe. Inevitably, these fragmented parts of the mind boomerang, as if inserted within the mind by a powerful outside force or a person, plotting to destroy or undermine peace of mind and sanity.

At the same time, a healthy part of the mind usually remains free of this process, and continues to give insight into distortions and paranoid thinking with a more balanced viewpoint. But if this healthy part of the mind is weakened for any reason, then distorted thinking may take over completely and lead to severe mental illness.

If feelings continue to intensify, blurring and confusion of thinking also develops within the important boundary area of 'self' and 'others'. As emotional pressures increase, the patient feels the boundary area around him is weakened or shattered. He may feel as if he has been perforated by the thoughts of others, that he is being hypnotised, no longer in charge of his mind. There is confusion about what is truly 'self' and what has been falsely put inside him by 'others'.

Changes of mood occur, and excitable inflated feelings take-over the stability of the mind with a 'high' of mood. Elation or manic behaviour may last for a period of days or weeks, although it is often short-lived, usually followed by a trough of guilt and depression.

Psychosis occurs when there is a complete break with reality, including all contact and relationships with others. In an attempt to find safety and security from the fragmentation process, there may be a withdrawal of the total personality within its own delusional (or severely distorted) psychological compartment, leading to isolation, loneliness and further distortion.

Visual and auditory hallucinations occur as thoughts and feelings become separate from the co-ordinating (ego) part of the mind, as if originating outside the body, rather than from within.

If you are experiencing a psychotic (break with reality) illness, you are quite likely to feel controlled by others, convinced that it is **'their'** thoughts, ideas, feelings, and motivating influences which causes your exhaustion, sense of confusion and the changes which are happening to your body and mind.

Remember that all psychological symptoms are aggravated by fatigue, impaired general health, drugs of abuse, alcohol, poor nutrition, strain, or any form of extreme psychological pressure. For this reason, try to keep these minimal.

7 Upper Harley Street
London NW1

HOMOEOPATHY AND PSYCHOLOGICAL ILLNESS

Homoeopathy acts deeply upon the mind, helping to loosen rigid defensive patterns of thinking and releasing blocked areas of repression. These include emotions and memories, together with their intrinsic energy, which in the past have undermined physical health and drained energy reserves.

It acts to restore order and balance, loosening emotional knots or 'no-go' areas within the mind, helping to recall and free past traumas and hurts to the conscious memory. They can then be thought about in a different, more balanced mature way. The homoeopathic potency can also liberate a spontaneous expression of feelings, allowing healthier relationships to flourish and grow. It supports the ability to openly acknowledge love, caring, and need, as well as hurts which were often denied in the past.

The homoeopathic approach promotes relaxation by reducing tension and treating it's fundamental cause. It promotes a rhythmic approach to life, rebuilding vital energy reserves and encouraging a relaxed frame of mind. It helps restore the sleep rhythm, as the mind becomes less active at night.

As tension and irritability are reduced, problems can be more easily discussed and resolved. This leads to the possibility of new insights developing, a lessening of negative self-destructive guilt, encouraging balanced judgements and greater confidence.

It is also helpful for the prevention and treatment of psychological illness, of value in puerperal (post-childbirth) psychosis, or where a depressive breakdown is feared. Here the patient is usually under great strain and pressure or there is a history of past depression.

Homoeopathy improves perspectives, reducing tension and anxiety levels, calming phobic fears and restores balance. It helps bring any underlying anguish or discord, memories and associations, back to the surface. In this way, they can become integrated into a more meaningful whole and a less distorted emotional approach to life.

The method is of value in manic-depressive illness, helping to reverse the psychotic process, restoring peace of mind and lessening sudden mood swings from elation to suicidal preoccupation.

Homoeopathy plays an important role in obsessional states and rigid patterns of behaviour, making them more amenable to counselling and psychotherapy, reducing the need for high or prolonged doses of conventional drugs which may cause side-effects.

By increasing an awareness of the workings of the mind, homoeopathy helps develop insights into distorted attitudes. In this way, previous insecurities and distorted viewpoints or attitudes can be changed and matured.

Your homoeopathic doctor will assess how the illness process is evolving and the strength and intensity of any mood changes. The remedies may need to be taken in much higher dilutions than the usual 6c or 30c strengths, possibly using a 200c strength or M potency.

A combination of homoeopathy and counselling is an ideal approach to psychological illness. When the illness is in an acute phase, distortions are often a major feature. These represent a form of psychological defence against hurt and rejection. At times, conventional remedies may be needed to contain the raw (instinctual) energy of some patients. But when homoeopathy is also used, conventional drugs may often be given in a reduced dosage. In many cases the drugs can be dispensed with altogether.

ADVICE ON TAKING HOMOEOPATHIC REMEDIES

Sources of remedies
The remedies recommended throughout the book should only be purchased directly from a homoeopathic pharmacy or health shop. Always ensure that your remedies are from a reliable source. Take them initially in the sixth (6c) strength, but use the stronger thirty (30c) potency if you fail to get an improvement.

Using the remedies
The potencies or strengths, come as small round pills or tablets, made of sucrose (or lactose). If you are sensitive to lactose, you should order your remedies directly from a homoeopathic pharmacy, requesting a sucrose or lactose-free pill base for the remedies. Because the medicine, or homoeopathic dilution is applied directly to the surface of the pill, they should not be handled. They are best placed directly into the mouth from the lid of the container, and sucked under the tongue. They should always be taken at least 20 minutes before or after food or drink (except water), orthodox medicines, vitamin or mineral supplements.

Substances to avoid
Do not drink peppermint tea when taking homoeopathic remedies. Avoid coffee, tea, and cocoa, because their high caffeine content may diminish their effect.

Keeping the remedies fresh and active
The medicines should be stored in a cool, dry, dark area, away from strong odours, especially camphor, oil of wintergreen, perfume, essential oils, after-shave, and soap. In this way, their action will last indefinitely.

Diet and alcohol

A bland diet is recommended, not eating to excess, or using strong spices. Alcohol should be avoided, and smoking reduced or stopped altogether during treatment, especially for lung, heart, or circulatory problems.

How long should remedies be taken for

Remedies should be taken for as long as symptoms persist, but stopped as soon as you are feeling better and the emotional symptoms have gone. If new symptoms arise during homoeopathic treatment, they should be watched carefully, especially if they have occurred in the past. The homoeopathic action may sometimes cause earlier symptoms to reappear. These are usually fleeting, but if persistent, they will require a new remedy.

Aggravation of symptoms

An aggravation of symptoms, after taking the remedies, is a positive sign and means the potencies are working well. It is usually short-lived, and does not undermine the overall sense of well-being and improved vitality.

Side-effects

If you use them correctly, there are no side-effects or risks from homoeopathy. If you take a wrong remedy, or a whole box of the pills, they will cause no harm. The remedies can be safely used during pregnancy and when breast-feeding, or given to the youngest baby.

Homoeopathy and orthodox medicines
The remedies do not interact with orthodox medicines, or undermine their action. If you are given a course of antibiotics, it is best to stop homoeopathic remedies until it is completed. Some orthodox drugs, especially oral steroids, may reduce or neutralise the homoeopathic effect.

Pain
Homoeopathy will help with some types of pain and spasm, but it is not the treatment of choice for very acute or severe pain and if this occurs, orthodox treatment is recommended.

Homoeopathy and the age of the patient
Homoeopathy acts at every age, the reaction varying with age, strength, and the intrinsic resistance or vital energy reserves of the patient. It acts very quickly in a child, or fit young person, but is slower in an elderly person, particularly if old, weak or feeble.

Homoeopathy and acute illness of the elderly
It is often better initially, to give an orthodox treatment to an elderly person during an acute illness. If possible, use homoeopathy when convalescent, and before severe weakness occurs.

Safety of the homoeopathic approach
Homoeopathy is helpful in the older age group, especially for muddled thinking, poor memory, insomnia, restlessness, anxiety or tension problems. It does not cause confusion of the mind or agitation, which may become a severe problem when some orthodox drugs are used.

AGITATION

Agitation of the mind is an overspill of pent-up tension and drive into the emotions, causing fidgety restlessness of body and mind. There is a sense of overwhelming energy, at times feeling like a pressure-cooker without a safety valve. An uneasy awareness of short-fuse energy may rock the whole body, as if every nerve is stretched, overloaded and shaking. The intensity of the energy release can cause spasm, pain, tension, tremor and strain of every joint and muscle fibre of the body from the jaw and scalp to the toe joints. There is a restless need to find relief from tension, sometimes pacing like a caged tiger, up and down, not knowing where to find rest or comfort. The emotional tension is equally powerful, churned up like a volcano about to erupt, and not finding comfort, peace or relaxation, from emotions which often cannot be easily expressed. The pressures may eventually undermine sleep, appetite, and all the normal elimination patterns of the body. Like the genie in the bottle, there seems no satisfactory way for the tension and feelings to find release.

The cause may not be immediately obvious. A thought may set off the agitation process, sometimes relating to insecurity, a past disappointment, a hurt, loss, or childhood incident. Sometimes another person, at home or work, is felt to pose a threat, or there is a change in routine, a shift in the status quo, the reassurance of a regular routine.

One patient became very agitated whenever her married daughter came to visit with the children. She liked to see them, but felt threatened, by having to make them a light meal, unable to cope with anything different from her usual set routine. In reality, her daughter always brought sandwiches, something simple to cook, and there was never a problem.

Agitation may be associated with severe depression, especially feelings of tension and inadequacy, causing early morning waking. The tension feels physical in origin, but the real problem is a frightening sense of losing control, not being able to cope, with fear of anger, violence, rejection or humiliation.

In the elderly it may be caused by any infection, with a raised temperature, sometimes high circulating levels of a particular pharmaceutical drug, especially a tranquilliser or sedative, but any drug given to excess, may cause agitation, especially those containing caffeine. In a similar way, high levels of coffee, cocoa, or tea, if taken to excess, may aggravate the problem.

Character traits which aggravate the condition
There is a tendency to panic, feel inadequate or easily defeated. Lack of confidence keeps feelings bottled up. At the least situation of uncertainty, they overspill as tension and agitation.

Practical steps to improve things
Try to relax before a crisis occurs. Broaden your experience with others and always discuss any doubts or anxieties you feel with your partner or family. De-fuse any tendency to accumulate anxiety which could lead to agitation, by discussing your feelings as soon as they occur. Try not to anticipate failure, or difficulty, but tackle each problem or new situation as it occurs, and always as a challenge rather than a disaster.

Remedies to consider:-

Aconitum   Indicated for very acute violent states of agitation, the face red and burning, the mood one of extreme fear and apprehension.

Arsenicum   A remedy where obsessional fears and anxiety is marked, the body ice cold and craving heat of any kind. There is a tendency to dislike closeness or company. Burning pains occur throughout the body, often worse after midnight.

Belladonna   The face is red, the body burning hot and dry, with high levels of fear and anxiety. Restlessness is marked.

Hyoscyamus   Agitation and tension are marked, with delusional beliefs. There is a tendency to suspicion or violence.

Stramonium   For problems of extreme agitation and excitement, the patient difficult to control and at times markedly overactive.

ALCOHOL-RELATED ILLNESS

Alcohol is one of the commonest social escapes from work or family problems and at the same time, one with the most potential for self-damage and destructive addiction. The habit is easy to acquire and often associated with depression, weakness, loss of confidence and a tendency to cover up problems rather than solve them or make fundamental changes.

Alcohol is a depressant, although initially there are pleasant feelings of warmth with an easing of tensions and inhibitions. Company and friends are made quickly, but the initial euphoria is soon followed by a low in mood, wanting to withdraw, and feelings of guilt or shame. Alcohol leads to loss of control, eventually allowing suspicion, jealousy, or fantasy to take over the personality. Reason and reality thinking may be temporarily lost, leading to misinterpretation of others, sometimes attacks of violence. But not everyone is aggressive, and some drinkers mellow, forget their problems for a time, become more assertive, and are able to relax. There is however a high price to be paid, in terms of physical well-being, with increased weight and a damaging effect upon the liver, stomach and cardiovascular system.

DELIRIUM TREMENS

This is an acute or sometimes chronic state of confusion due to alcoholic poisoning of the central nervous system. Because of depression of the brain and cortex, judgement and perception are affected. This undermines thought and the co-ordinating mechanisms, leading to visual hallucinations and a variety of misperceptions and misunderstanding which are mainly delusional in type. Physical problems are often the result of a degeneration of the peripheral nervous system. Neuritis occurs due to inflammation of the nerves of the hands and feet, which then tingle and twitch, or feel as if there is something moving and alive under the flesh.

Most movements are unreliable and accompanied by swaying movement or tremor. The stomach feels nauseated, or thick and distasteful, vision is uncertain, cloudy or blurred, due to retinal neuritis, and anxiety levels may be high. The only way to find relief is to take more alcohol, which gives a temporary feeling of respite from the symptoms. But more than one drink, may provoke further confusion, a staggering gait, and lisping speech.

Character traits which aggravate the condition
There is a profound insecurity problem, which is denied or temporarily obliterated by alcohol. The drink problem does not however lead to permanent solutions, and tends to worsen problems and creates more difficulties rather than resolving them.

Practical steps to improve things
Try to evolve a method of gaining control over the drink problem, or any other situation where you take flight into eating or drinking, either at work or in the home. Talk more openly and honestly, when you are not drinking. Take the family with you if you need a drink and don't drink alone. Always tell your partner what is annoying or worrying you, and try to find another way of coping with the extent of your feelings. Don't let emotions build up out of control so that they overwhelm you.

Remedies to consider:-

Aconitum
Indicated for acute alcohol related problems, the face red and burning, the temples pulsating. It is of especial value when there are major symptoms of restlessness and fear.

Arsenicum
Anxiety is marked with a restless depression and fear. Always chilly, he craves heat, even in midsummer. Burning pains are present, often associated with chronic digestion problems. He dislikes being alone, yet is worse for company or consolation. All symptoms are worse in the early night hours, especially between 1-3.00 am.

Avena sat
The major indication for this remedy is debility and exhaustion as a result of alcohol abuse. The limbs feel weak or numb, and concentration is poor.

Natrum mur
Indicated when the problem is linked to underlying anxiety and depression.

Nux vomica

An important medicine for chronic alcoholism due to stress. There are chronic indigestion problems, pain, flatulence and heartburn (the result of gastritis), and chronic constipation. Mood swings vary from depression to irritability.

Plumbum met

This remedy is particularly indicated when there are problems of neuritis, as a result of drinking. Sudden spasms of muscular pain occur, with cramps or paralysis of certain muscles in the hands or feet.

Silicea

Indicated where there is timidity and a need for 'dutch courage'.

Thuja

A remedy for chronic alcohol problems. There is weakness, and exhaustion, always feeling cold and chilly, never really fit and well. Many of the symptoms may have occurred following a vaccination.

ANOREXIA NERVOSA

This is essentially a problem of young adolescent women, but it may sometimes occur in men, and sometimes adults.

In nearly all those involved, there is underlying distortion of the body image causing a compulsion to diet and lose weight. Although the body may be thin to the point of being at starvation point, the weight down to five stones or less, the anorexic may still feel fat, bloated and unattractive, legs and thighs too big, hips wide, bottom obvious or protruding despite severe muscle wasting and loss of fat and protein (muscle). The whole pelvic area may in reality, look thin and almost skeletal. Menstruation usually ceases totally and it may be many years before the periods are re-established again.

Even when the patient is beginning to improve, there may be a preoccupation with increasing weight too quickly, or fear of losing her under-nourished look, anxiety at developing a stomach, but especially any shapely sexual characteristics - a bottom, 'front', thighs or hips. At the same time there is a paradoxical shame and dislike at being so obviously shapeless and thin, having to hide, fearful of comments when out shopping, at the pool, wearing a swimming costume.

Every anorexic experiences diametrically opposing feelings concerning her body shape and form. She wants to improve and be well, feel less tired, to feel warm, with a shape and form to her body, to have periods again and be less susceptible to colds, flu, illness. This contrasts with an overwhelming fear of change.

23

There is often anxiety about weight-gain, wanting to improve, yet at the same time, insistent that any changes are slow (really under her own control).

Anorexia is often associated with bulimia, or bingeing followed by compulsive self-induced vomiting, picking at food, eating only minute low calorie meals. Mood swings occur with excessive nervous energy, only to be followed by exhaustion and total collapse. There is a tendency to stimulate regurgitation vomiting after eating, to deny feelings of rage, frustration, boredom, loneliness, fear and often despair.

Character traits which aggravate the condition
The anorexic is often intolerant, fussy and perfectionistic. Everything must be in order and under control, leading to a pressurised mentality (stemming from an over-strict demanding conscience) which dislikes untidiness, disorder, imperfection or mess.

Practical steps to improve things
Try to be more tolerant, less rigid and fixed in your attitudes. Expect that every person and situation will be different and aim to respond to these with different aspects of yourself, in this way becoming more flexible. Widen your social experiences, with a broader group of interests and people. Avoid keeping to a single narrow relationship which is unsatisfactory or frustrating, and where you are unable to give of yourself or find happiness. Explore as many new situations as possible, but at the same time, find something which you are good at, enjoy and can develop in greater depth. If you feel frustrated or angry, avoid taking it out on your body by bingeing or vomiting. Talk openly about any problems. Express anger as well as love and affection.

Remedies to consider:-

Argentum nit   There are high levels of phobic anxiety, avoiding shops, busy centres and contacts with new people. Intolerance of heat.

Arsenicum   Always chilly and cold, the main problem is severe agitation and anxiety, often quite severe depression. Many symptoms are worse in the early night hours, especially after midnight.

Natrum mur   A remedy for profound states of insecurity and inadequacy, never at ease socially and avoiding close contact with others. Fear and weakness are worse for consolation or sympathy. Salt is craved.

Phosphorus   For mild cases of anorexia, with a weak chest and often asthma. She is chilly and always cold, yet craves cold drinks. There is a constant searching for attention and reassurance.

Tuberculinum   There is a severe weight loss, a restless temperament, always on the move and unable to relax. A recurrent nervous dry cough is characteristic.

ANXIETY STATES

Depending upon the extent of work or family pressures and problems, some degree of anxiety is normal and unavoidable. Usually this only becomes an illness, when very high levels of tension are sustained over a prolonged period, undermining rest and relaxation. For many, once a problem has been resolved, anxiety symptoms may disappear almost entirely, sometimes for months or years. They may however reappear at times of extreme strain:- following a loss, after a new baby, when made redundant, an illness of a member of the family, or during the break-up of a relationship. The major manifestation of anxiety is severe and prolonged tension or fear, which is inappropriate to the present situation. The mind is in a state of turmoil or panic, as an excess of anxiety threatens to take over relaxation, sleep, and peace of mind.

If the emotions are pushed down, to prevent them getting out of control, they may overspill into the autonomic nervous system which controls the major physiological processes, creating unpleasant symptoms of overactivity and stress in these areas. The heart may feel disagreeably full, beat strongly and quickly, with palpitations and a heightened awareness of its pumping action. The bladder becomes irritated, the bowels react with diarrhoea, or sometimes constipation, the appetite and digestion also affected, with nausea, acidity, flatulence, heartburn and colic.

As the emotional tension rises, energy levels also increase, anticipating either flight or a conflict situation. Adrenalin release leads to increased muscular tension, releasing waves of heat as sweat, the whole body trembling and bathed in sweat. Other symptoms include:- a 'lump' in the throat, restless tremor, shaking fits, insomnia, nervous laughter or tears, hoarseness, an irritating dry cough, eczema, shortness of breath, sighing breathing, an empty dragging-down sensation in the pit of the stomach, as energy is depleted by the strength of emotions. There may also be an increased susceptibility to infection with recurrent colds, as vitality and reserves are drained away.

Character traits which aggravate the condition

There is a tendency to over-react to new situations and a damaging tendency to keep feelings and emotions buried or controlled. This is mainly due to fear of any sudden surge of emotion or losing control. Spontaneity is limited or absent and security and trust tends to be low. There has often been damage in early childhood, occurring at the time of a major psychological phase of exploration and growth.

Practical steps to improve things

Aim to be easy, open and spontaneous with others, especially with new friends and in new situations. Try to let your feelings out and say what you feel at the time. Don't be inhibited by fear of embarrassment or losing control. Clarify any childhood aspects of behaviour which you think may still be perpetuating, the anxiety problems and slowly aim to correct these by more varied social experiences. Trust yourself more and allow your natural gifts and interests to develop. Remember, you don't have to be mainstream in all your beliefs and interests. Breaking with conformity, conditioning, and tradition is often an advantage, a sign of more creative thinking.

Remedies to consider:-

Aconitum

Indicated for acute and recent anxiety problems with fear and agitation.

Argentum nit

For severe anticipatory anxiety, especially when travelling away from home or appearing in public. Intolerance of heat.

Arsenicum

Agitation, apprehension and irritability are marked, keeping others at a distance. There is extreme fatigue and obsessional mannerisms, such as neatness. Quickly irritable and depressed, he is a loner in temperament.

Gelsemium

A useful remedy for hysterical or dramatic forms of anxiety when there are many attachments to the past. An identification with parental ideals is often a defence against being more assertive and independent in the present. Confidence levels are low.

Natrum mur

For tense, fearful, anxious states, never at ease with others or in any social situation. He tends to feel worse for sympathy or consolation.

Nux vomica   There is an irritable state of mind, with spasms of short-fuse anger, and a temperament which is far too anxious and intolerant.

Phosphorus   For the fearful, insecure person who functions in flashes of short-lasting energy and drive. There is a constant need for reassurance that he is liked and approved of.

Sepia   A remedy for complaining, negative depressive anxiety, accompanied by fatigue and indifference. All symptoms are worse at the end of the day, but better for vigorous exercise, especially from dancing.

Silicea   A major remedy where anxiety is associated with lack of drive, fear of failure, with physical and psychological weakness in many different situations. Withdrawal and lack of competitive spirit are other indications for this remedy.

CONFIDENCE LOSS

Confidence occurs at an early stage of development, fostered by a close bonding relationship between infant and mother. Unless the delivery or the pregnancy has been traumatic, precipitate or excessively painful, associated with a separation, confidence is a natural outcome of this trust, and present from birth. It can be clearly seen in the confident way the young baby takes the breast or bottle, the way he moves, grabs, sucks, cries, kicks, screams, and holds. The confident child is spontaneous and direct. Unless this process is interfered with by an over-anxious mother or some other form of emotional damage, abuse, or trauma, it continues to grow and forms the foundation-stone of adult confidence, strength and the ability to deal with people and situations, to feel free and at ease with both self and others.

Loss of confidence causes fear, anticipation of rejection, anxiety about loss of love or approval. Hesitancy rather than spontaneity and directness becomes the norm, with a tendency to hold-back, to be self-critical, anticipate disasters or expect failure, often feeling inferior to others and a second class citizen. There may be a quite overwhelming terror of new situations and relationships, or any form of physical or psychological closeness.

Where there is a moderate loss of confidence, the causes are often obvious, requiring common sense action with support and caring reassurance from friends and members of the family.

Severe loss of confidence, gives rise to much higher levels of fear, feeling exposed, or at a disadvantage in some way, reactivating infantile fears of rejection, sometimes a lost or small feeling, as if trapped in a corner of life and fearing to come out. It is common to feel that any form of admission of feelings of need and closer contact with others, will inevitably lead to being stared or laughed at. This is usually due to embarrassment or an over critical conscience (demanding perfection at every stage of life), with guilt feelings about not having been more assertive, giving or demonstrably loving in the past.

Character traits which aggravate the condition

There is a damaging tendency to withdraw from angry disputes and strong feelings, because of the intensity of the feelings. But avoiding any confrontation or challenge, eventually leads to weakness and loss of confidence. Withdrawal into the self further undermines confidence and social experience.

Practical steps to improve things

Begin by deciding to assert yourself openly, to be less apologetic in your relationship with others. Try to curb any tendency to withhold and deny feelings or ideas and give every aspect of yourself a greater chance to evolve and develop. If you have experienced a hurt in the past, don't allow yourself to become dominated by it and try to build upon it. If you allow yourself to be pressurised in this way, you are really evading the present and giving in to a form of psychological self-abuse and bullying, albeit your own anger and resentment. It is destructive to think only about the past, when what really matters is how you act and are today.

Remedies to consider:-

Argentum nit

For confidence loss of a phobic kind, with a tendency to keep to a narrow area of safety close to the home. If this is extended in any way, panic attacks may occur due to insecurity and fear. There is intolerance of heat.

Calcarea

Insecurity is marked, lacking energy and drive. There is a tendency to withdraw into fantasy, often with obsessional preoccupations of a repetitive type.

Gelsemium

For hysterical (dramatic) states of mind. There are usually strong dependant ties to the family, and infantile attitudes which dominate all aspects of mature adult behaviour. Fear of talking in public is a common problem.

Lycopodium

A useful remedy for lack of confidence and underlying insecurity in a person who gives the impression of being mature and able to cope. He talks well, but is rarely at ease with his own peer group. Everything in life is clumsy, rushed, precipitate and off balance, causing a weak base for security and confidence.

Natrum mur

Recommended when there is a lack of ease, rarely relaxed with others and worse for close social contacts or sympathy. The lack of confidence is accompanied by a weeping depression and feelings of exhaustion.

Pulsatilla

A remedy for variable, changing moods, which create an unstable psychological platform for relationships with others. Emotions vary from one moment or situation to another, causing a sense of vulnerability. He is rarely ever fully relaxed or able to enjoy life. A series of dramatic situations causes exhaustion and a sense of being out of control. Psychological manipulation of others is common.

Silicea

Weakness, lack of drive, fear of failure, apprehension, undermine health and confidence. This is further drained by a debilitating series of physical illnesses, usually due to recurrent infection.

33

CONFUSIONAL STATES

When the mind becomes confused, it is often the result of withdrawal, and fudging the difference (or boundary), between self and others, fantasy and reality. It may become impossible to function in a clear appropriate way, because judgment and perception are dominated by impulse and fantasy, both of which take their basic assumptions about reality from the inner imaginative world of the mind rather than outer reality. The safe haven of the inner world, because it blurs and distorts, is mainly preoccupied with narcissistic (self-directed) fantasies. This creates problems of understanding and relating to others, often difficulty in making sense of what is happening in the world of reality, causing misunderstanding and loss of trust.

The reason for confusion may sometimes be physical, often due to an acute infection associated with a high temperature. Other examples are the side-effects of a particular drug, prescribed in too a high dose for the needs of the individual.

Confusion may also occur during the course of any acute psychological illness, as an expression of fear and flight from a disturbed and distorted picture of reality. It is particularly common in psychotic states, when fragmentation of the logical thought processes creates terrifying fantasy imagery, which becomes confused with reality. But it may also occur during profound periods of depression, as part of an acute anxiety state or as a manifestation of hysteria. Psychological illness of the elderly often first manifests as acute confusion, with misperception of others and paranoid thinking.

Character traits which aggravate the condition
There is a tendency to be rigid or fixed in attitudes and thinking. Obsessional character traits, may occur with undue emphasis on order and routine, at the same time feeling vulnerable and de-personalised in a new or strange environment. There is usually dislike of change, new people or new situations, and these are felt to pose a threat. The problem of change and adjustment tends to become worse as the person gets older.

Practical steps to improve things
You may not always be aware of becoming confused in a familiar setting, and with close members of the family your mind may be absolutely clear. If you feel under pressure, your thinking fuzzed, your head about to explode with thoughts which will not turn off and let you relax, always discuss the feelings as soon as they occur, with a friend or member of the family. Also try to describe any feelings of being the object of a campaign to annoy or provoke you in any way. If you are taking a prescribed drug from your doctor, and feel that your mind will not wind down or stop, like an overwound clock, then discuss this with him and the possibility that you are reacting to one of your drugs. The best way to minimise confusion is to talk about it as soon as the feelings come up. If sleep is affected, you are restless at night, unable to sleep or rest during the day, discuss this with your doctor as early as possible. Try to be regular and rhythmic throughout the day, pacing yourself physically and emotionally, so that you do not over-react or exhaust yourself in social or family relationships.

Remedies to consider:-

Belladonna

The face is red or livid, hot, pupils dilated, neck and temple arteries pulsating strongly. The mood is one of excitement and strain, to the point of rage or fury. Because of a confusional state of mind, there are many fears and imaginative ideas. He feels unreal, at times in a dream-like state. There is intolerance of bright lights and noise.

Hyoscyamus

For hyper-excitable manic states, with confusion and violence. Speech is frequently incoherent, the words used disconnected or inappropriate. There is a high level of anxiety, causing a variety of contrasting moods, constantly talking, dancing, raving, hitting out at others, laughing, forgetful, with everything done in a hurry. Because of the confusion, he may not recognize his own family.

Opium

There is a mood of confusion and rage, the face red, eyes glistening. Moods vary, at times he is overactive, fearful of animals or other small objects. Fear of impending death causes him to weep or cringe, to feel terrified, weak, exhausted. At times he is

36

brighter and more energetic, at other times, almost comatose. Concentration is poor and he is forgetful, with a tendency to lie or falsify. There are frequently problems of very severe constipation.

Pulsatilla

A remedy for anxious, confused, variable states of mind. Many symptoms are worse at night, and from heat, but improved with fresh air. The mood is often hypochondriacal, depressed, and pessimistic. Uncertainty and lack of confidence, leads him to keep changing his mind. He is often tearful and always in a hurry. He is fearful and ill at ease with the opposite sex, often dominated by compulsive thoughts of death or drowning. Chronic nasal or sinus congestion is typical, also venous congestion, with liver complaints, piles or varicose veins. There is a tendency to flush up easily and an absence of thirst.

Stramonium

A remedy for wild, excitable, irrational hyper-manic states of mind. He is quickly confused, with muddled thinking and ideas, using wrong words or names, making spelling mistakes. The memory is usually poor. The face

is often red and flushed. At times
he may develop a withdrawn,
comatose or stupefied state of
mind, impossible to communicate
with. He has an abject dread of
all fluids, especially water, and
even thinking about it may cause
a crisis of nerves.

Sulphur

A deep-acting remedy for
debilitated, irritable, changing,
vague states of mind. He is often
depressed, worse on waking and
in the evening. Nothing is ever
fully enjoyed, and he suffers from
burning discomfort:- in the chest,
stomach, rectum, on passing
water, but at the same time, the
limbs feel cold due to poor
circulation. All his ideas are
vague, speculative, and
philosophical, his memory
unreliable, and he often cannot
relate ideas together in a sensible
way. He is often insensitive to the
feelings of others, giving his ideas
and thoughts an exaggerated
importance. There are chronic
bowel problems, waking with an
offensive diarrhoea which drives
him from the bed. His appearance
is dirty and neglected, the skin
infected, and he dislikes both
water and washing.

DELUSIONS

Delusions are a form of misperception of the external world, the result of distortion of reality, by fear, suspicion, and fantasy. Mistrust and malice occur as a feature of everyday imaginative thinking, with omnipotent fantasies of either abounding love or destructiveness, sometimes involving sexual control and possessiveness, usually only briefly known about in flashes of recalled dreams. But in a delusional state, these unconscious themes dominate waking life, creating distortions in the waking world, so that others are felt to be all-powerful, evil, or at times weak and vulnerable.

An acute delusional state may be due to poisoning by a variety of toxic substances, including poisonous plants or fungi, excess alcohol, drugs of abuse (especially LSD), sometimes prescribed drugs, for example when given in high doses to an elderly patient, during any acute physical illness with a high temperature, such as tonsillitis or meningitis, or the result of senility. Delusional states sometimes occur because of a brain tumour, or follow a head injury with concussion and brain damage, or after an acute and catastrophic industrial accident (e.g. the loss of a limb).

The most common cause of a delusional state, is of emotional origin, due to an acute psychotic (break with reality) state of mind, with fragmentation of both thought and feelings. This may have followed an acute shock, loss, disappointment, or rejection, or occurred slowly and insidiously over a period of years. In many cases, the cause is not obvious and the events which lead to the psychotic process are not clear, or spoken about. Often they are subtle and relate to tensions within the family dynamics, often an unhappy childhood, or marriage, sometimes both. Over a period of years, the patient may have been the psychological recipient of all the stress and tension currents which existed within the family. He may have been labelled as the problem, shy, ill, or limiting member who caused all their problems and difficulties, and then become resented or rejected. This may have led to damaging overprotective or suppressive attitudes towards all forms of spontaneous self-expression and sexuality.

Typical delusional symptoms include:- feelings of persecution, being stared at, picked upon, talked about, or discriminated in some way. Often this has a reality base, but becomes exaggerated out of all proportion. A particular object may be missing and cannot be found, perhaps an unusual noise is given undue prominence and attention. There is often fear of, as well as the need for, interest and attention, and being singled out for attention, even in a paranoid persecutory way, implies being special, unique and noticed. In many ways, this may be preferable to indifference or being ignored, because of underlying loss of self-confidence and low self-esteem.

Character traits which aggravate the condition

The problem is often caused by rigid controlling attitudes, a tendency to be passive, to look at and watch others, or to listen to them without comment, or declaring underlying feelings of anger and frustration. For some, the origins are rooted in infancy, when any loud or spontaneous comment was disapproved of and the child was made to be seen, but not heard. Physical punishment in childhood may have worsened the delusional tendency, by stimulating destructive fantasies and violence and at the same time repressing them.

Practical steps to improve things

Talk to your partner about any intense feelings of anger or rage, caring and need, as you experience them, even if the feelings date back many years. If you feel irritable and incensed, then talk about it, and find a creative outlet for this kind of energy, perhaps through art or music, in the home or garden. Try to build on these feelings, always staying in touch with reality, but at the same time allowing any early memories and feelings to be expressed. But don't allow them to dominate or take over. Try writing a story about them, perhaps a play, but use the energy positively and give it a shape and an end-result in the present rather than allowing it to turn in upon yourself, which is ultimately a self-destructive process. Exercise regularly, and make time for daily relaxation, if necessary using a relaxation tape, meditation, or yoga.

Remedies to consider:-

Argentum nit

A remedy for delusional beliefs accompanied by hallucinations, usually of a phobic type. He is intolerant of heat, the memory poor, and with an overwhelming sense of fatigue. Irritable, he is always in a hurry and erratic. The deluded state of mind may lead to self-destructive impulses to throw himself from a tall building into water. Other bizarre ideas relate to a distortion of the body image, with a sense of expansion of one limb, or throughout the body.

Belladonna

Delusional beliefs are expressed forcibly through a hyper-excitable state of body and mind. During this state of mind, the face is red and feels hot, the pupils dilated. There are many delusional beliefs which involve animals, especially dogs, but also insects and other small objects, which swarm over him in a threatening way. The face may feel transparent and he has many terrifying hallucinations of ghosts and phantoms. At times muscular excitability leads to peculiar spasms or contractions. He is over-sensitive to light, noise, touch and odour.

Cannabis ind   Indicated for confused excitable states of mind, where there are vivid, fixed delusional ideas. He feels as if he is about to die, that people are plotting to kill him or is convinced he can fly. He may feel persecuted and attacked by demons. At other times he feels divided, one part looking down upon himself from a great height. The mood is usually one of elation and over-talkativeness. Concentration is poor, because ideas and associations flood into his mind. Time is felt to pass too slowly and each minute may seem like a year or a lifetime.

Cocculus   There is a confused, deluded state of mind, marked by severe anxiety and wild mood swings. Time passes too quickly, and he feels a mixture of paralytic weakness or exhaustion and also irritability. There is often a sense of void or emptiness. He is remote and withdrawn, all ideas and rational thoughts seem to be in a vacuum. He finds words difficult to express himself with, and he may eventually become immobile or sit staring silently into space.

Ignatia

The delusional psychotic illness is often provoked by an acute (recent) loss, grief or disappointment. He is usually cut-off from reality, full of self-destructive pessimistic ideas and guilt feelings, as if he has committed a crime. He sees every aspect of life as a disaster. Anxious, irritable, and extremely hypersensitive, he is impatient, with rapid mood changes. At other times he is depressed and quiet, but quickly changing to laughter, then tears.

Hyoscyamus

A remedy for violent, hyper-manic, delusional, destructive states of mind. He is confused, hearing voices and tries to escape, preoccupied with distorted, unreal ideas and thinking. At times he acts inappropriately, with odd gestures or sudden mood swings, laughing to himself, or at the voices he hears in his head. There are also impulses to bite or strike out at others. Fear of water is a major source of anxiety. Suspicious, he sees images which threaten him, or believes others are plotting against him, or he is being poisoned.

Lachesis   There is a hyper-active, over-talkative state of mind. He is irritable and excitable, with alternating moods of depression and agitation. Arrogant and proud, at times he is mistrustful and jealous. He is frequently irritable and quick to anger. All forms of tight or restrictive clothing are avoided, aggravating any symptoms. Exhaustion is marked, at the same time as over-activity. He has paranoid delusional ideas of a plot to detain or imprison him, or believes he is already dead, living in a dream world, convinced he is about to die. Religious ideas may dominate his thinking, believing he has committed an unpardonable sin and will go directly to hell or damnation. At other times he feels under the influence of supernatural powers. All the symptoms are worse after sleep.

Petroleum   The mood is one of variable excitement, quick to anger or violence. He is hypochondriacal, with no drive or will-power. Hypersensitive, the least thing can provoke or cause him to fly into a rage. Memory is poor, and he quickly loses his way, even in familiar situations. He is

45

convinced that death is quite imminent and feels he must put his affairs in order. At other times, he seems split or double, as if another person is lying beside him. There is a profound sense of exhaustion, feeling chilly and hungry, the stomach empty. The skin is dry or irritated, often infected and cracking.

Phosphoric acid   This remedy is indicated for lively exaggerated states of mood. At times, he is tearful or depressed, and then becomes quiet and indifferent. He is apathetic and exhausted mentally and physically, lacking the strength to express himself clearly.

Sabadilla   He is quick to anger and to violence. The delusional beliefs may lead to feelings that his body has shrunk in size, turned into a corpse, the stomach corroded. Other parts feel swollen, e.g. the testicles feel enlarged. The limbs may feel twisted or shortened, the chin elongated, bigger on one side of the face than the other. He is excessively hypochondriacal. Moods are variable, excitable or depressed. The mind and thought processes are slowed down.

46

Thuja

He imagines his body is make of glass and is terrified in case it fragments into pieces.

Stramonium

For violent, restless, noisy, deluded states of mind. He sees danger at every corner of life and fears being attacked by dogs. There are hyper-manic mood swings, leading to uncontrollable destructive behaviour. At times he is full of fear and sees insects coming at him. The pupils are typically dilated. There is an aversion to liquids of any kind, and giving water to drink may cause an acute spasm or contraction of the mouth, or stiffening of the whole body. All movements are quick and clumsy. The body image is distorted, with a sense of being elongated, pulled out, or extended.

Sulphur

There is an anxious, confused state of mind. He tends to be irritable and violent, full of unrelated ideas and thoughts, the speech disjointed and nonsensical. He fears he has neglected his work or business or that others have injured him in some way and will cause his death. The mood is despondent and pessimistic. At the same time he idealises vague speculative ideas. Even rags are beautiful. The head and entire body feels burning hot, but the feet are ice cold. All symptoms are worse for heat and contact with water or washing. The digestive system is usually chronically upset with severe problems of flatulence, wind and heartburn. He may be driven out of bed on waking by an offensive diarrhoea. The skin is typically infected with a chronic eczema, or individual spots which ooze or discharge pus.

DEPRESSION

At times everyone feels 'down in the dumps' that it is not worth the effort, a failure, unappreciated and unwanted or that fate is against them. These are usually fleeting doubts, which are quite normal. In a depressive psychological illness, emotions are much more intense and deep; feelings are swamped or overwhelmed by a profound depth of despair and anguish. There is a lack of hope, belief or confidence, in both self and the future. A black, gloomy, flattening negative mood may pervade everything from the moment of first waking.

The whole day may be affected by this mood of despair, often beginning in the early morning hours, and sometimes lasting for weeks or months. Drive and energy are reduced by a conviction of failure, often feeling defeated by life and quite simple events, leading to a downward spiral of hopelessness, whatever the realities of the 'problem' or situation. Sleep is undermined, because of difficulty in getting off to sleep, which is often restless and shallow, or filled with dreams or nightmares. Early waking is a common feature, wide awake at 5.00 a.m. or earlier, feeling tired and wretched, with 'butterflies in the stomach' (due to tension), sometimes dreading having to face another day.

The cause is not always clear, but depression often originates from an early infantile or childhood emotional trauma, particularly a rejection, or it may relate to insecurity caused by lack of understanding or separation of the parents at a critical time of development. Verbal or physical abuse by a parent, sibling, half-brother, step-parent, grandparent, or teacher may have occurred at an early stage in development, causing damage and accumulated resentment. The death of a parent or a sibling, the loss of a much loved pet are other common causes of depression, usually associated with guilt feelings. In others, a suicide, the accidental death of a parent, departure of a 'nanny', leads to profound feelings of being unloved and abandoned, a sense of loneliness and despair which persists throughout life. Others are depressed because of grieving for a lost brother or sister they never knew. The mother may have miscarried at an age, when there was a profound longing for a sibling, not to feel alone and rootless. But such feelings are also ambivalent, with fear of being pushed out or displaced, leading to a sense of guilt and depression in later years.

Character traits which aggravate the condition

There is a tendency to live in the past, to feel guilty or responsible for the hurts of others. A close parental attachment, may be present, even in later life, albeit disapproving and critical, leading to feelings of resentment or rage about being too easily influenced, or moulded by parental values and ideals in the past. Such feelings tend to block any balancing sense of appreciation, love and gratitude for what is possible and acceptable. Living in the past, keeps you emotionally immature and limited, as if in a restrictive 'corner' of life, rather than in the centre ground of things as they happen. It is important to feel more involved, a part of life and less fearful, reaching out towards others, taking part, giving and receiving.

Practical steps to improve things

Try to become involved with others, spontaneous with every part of **you**, including speech, gestures, movement, reaching out, giving to others, showing how much you really care, appreciate, and can respond. Aim to be flexible and easy in your interests. Travel, looking and seeing, allowing yourself unrestricted and varied experiences. Maximise all your interests and contacts. If you feel infantile and frightened, then admit these feelings, and allow these fragile and vulnerable, child-like parts of yourself, into the 'room' (your contacts and relationships with others). Don't exclude any feelings or fears you may have, but acknowledge and admit them, allowing them to become part of you, loved and accepted, and not pushed out, nor just tolerated or resented. Talk and communicate with these primitive, infantile, needing, but often frightening aspects of yourself, and try not to deny them or push them into a corner where they can be ignored. If you find yourself particularly depressed, try making contact with these infantile and needing feelings, and find out from them what has triggered your depression and why. Don't laugh at, feel embarrassed by, or reject these emerging aspects of yourself. Try to reach out and encourage them to be known by you, rather than denying or devaluing them, because this will again be damaging and undermine your growth and confidence.

Remedies to consider:-

Arsenicum

There is suicidal despair with anguish and restless feelings, worse from 1.00-3.00 am. Weeps with a sense of hopelessness. Fear of death, confused, indifferent to life and others. Always chilly, usually thin and sweats. He is a loner and feels worse for reassurance or social contacts with others. Weakness is marked, also burning sensations in the body. He is always better for heat. There are many obsessional features which dominate thinking.

Aurum met

The depression is profound with a melancholic hopeless feeling of failure and having no future. Suicidal thoughts dominate all thinking, and there may be a history of a previous overdose. Joint rheumatic or arthritic pains, also palpitations add to the misery and the despair.

Calcarea

Typically fair, flabby, pale, and always chilly, tending to sweat on the head and face. Tired and exhausted, he is depressed, obsessional, and irritable with everything and everyone. Irritability is a marked feature, also palpitations.

52

Chelidonium

There is sadness with weeping, also anxiety and depression. He is apathetic, lacking drive and energy, but at the same time easily becoming irritable with mood swings.

China

For depression with feelings of exhaustion and no energy reserves. Mood swings vary from excitability to black irritable suicidal despair. He is a loner and at times has no desire to live, silent, indifferent, and hypochondriacal. Extreme flatulence is a common problem.

Ferrum met

There is a gloomy depression with exhaustion, feeling anxious, fearful and pessimistic. He expects some dreadful evil to happen to him at any moment, and this contributes to his short-fuse irritability. Weakness, hot flushes, palpitations, shortness of breath, may occur, worse after resting, and all symptoms are aggravated by noise.

Graphites

There is weeping despair with severe depression and thoughts of death. Anxious, irritable, timid and apprehensive. Everything seems to offend him or leads to an angry outburst. Fear of death dominates much of the thinking, and he is always extremely sensitive, worsening the fears. Music often leads to increased anxiety and to tears.

Lilium tig   A remedy for a weeping, fearful, apprehensive form of depression. At times he is timid, but he can become violently irritable, worse for consolation or any close social contact. Concentration is weak, and he finds difficulty in finding words or expressing himself clearly. Agitation is a marked feature and he is always in a hurry.

Lycopodium   Depression is caused by panic, especially anxiety about the future, lacking confidence and always poised for flight from any new challenging situation. He constantly anticipates failure and is easily put off trying to work or compete. At the same time he is quick, impetuous, accident-prone and often the centre of a risky game or project. He is limited by always wanting to rush ahead, and this undermines concentration and success. He rarely stays long enough in any one situation to give himself the foundations needed to build up confidence and experience. Basically a loner, he prefers some company in the house, but makes little real meaningful contact. He usually appears more confident and mature than he is in reality.

Medusa

This is mainly a remedy for adolescent depressive problems, the youth sulky and silent, or withdrawn and uninterested in making contact with others.

Natrum arsen

For a depressed, gloomy sense of impending disaster, irritable and silent. He always feels cold, often weak, and is usually underweight.

Natrum mur

A remedy for depression with profuse weeping, chilly and cold, thin, bent over with problems and difficulties. He is worse for consolation, or any social contacts and prefers to be alone. The depression has usually taken over the whole of the personality with a sense of disappointment. Mood changes are frequent and he is often worried about health. Oversensitive, he is usually worse for sea air, and craves salt.

Natrum sulph   Indicated for a silent, often severe suicidal form of depression with irritability. He is aggravated by music, and frequently feels worse on waking, with early morning anguish. Confidence levels are low and he is convinced that all attempts will end in failure. Oversensitivity further limits drive and confidence. Concentration levels are low. He constantly fears loss of control or madness.

Platina   This remedy is indicated for irritable states of mind. There is a marked sense of pride and an arrogant superiority, looking down upon others as small and insignificant, yet at the same time feeling depressed and restless. Fear of death, or anxiety when alone are signs of the underlying lack of confidence. Constricting pains are characteristic, like a tight band, especially around the head.

Pulsatilla   A remedy for variable states of tearful depression, with mood swings, and a timid disposition constantly seeking reassurance. Self-confidence and assertiveness are weak. There is an intolerance of heat, lack of thirst, and an intense dislike of fats.

Psorinum

A very useful remedy for unhappy, fearful, complaining states of depression, oppressed by a sense of anguish, fearing death or business failure. He weeps constantly but can also be very irritable and self-willed, insensitive to the feelings and needs of others. Irritability occurs with the depressive moods, also palpitations. Memory is poor. A chronic skin infection is frequently present, dirty or grey-looking and discharging pus.

Sepia

A remedy for an irritable type of depression with feelings of indifference to the family and those closest and most needed. There is a negative attitude to any suggestions, dragged down by fatigue and anguish, like a heavy weight. There is loss of libido, waking early, depressed and apathetic. The least display of reassurance or consolation leads to resentment. A dragging down low back pain is common, combined with exhaustion and despair. When the depression involves a woman at the menopause, heavy flooding with clots may occur. The male is irritable and intolerant, with recurrent abdominal or back pain.

DIET AND NUTRITION

The ideal diet for stress is balanced sensible eating. Any form of experimentation with dieting for a few weeks and then changing again, creates extra pressure and is undesirable. Eating balanced, healthy, sensible meals should be a way of life. Your food should be varied throughout the year, according to your mood and needs, as well as the seasons. Don't force yourself to eat if you don't feel like it or you are not hungry and avoid eating just for the sake of it. Heavy or unnecessary meals cause a jaded sense of fatigue and this adds to any lack of energy or drive from psychological causes. But however you feel, always eat healthy fresh food every day, if possible picked from your own garden, allotment, or your local farm shop, to ensure that what you put into your system contains minimal pesticide residues, and is preferably organically grown. Quick, pre-cooked, or microwaved foods should be avoided.

Eat slowly, without rushing and with appreciation. Aim to feel some sense of reverence, always aware that a great deal of your food is a living thing. More time should be given to meals, how they are presented and prepared. They are important times within the day, and often social occasions, sharing thoughts and feelings, also quiet moments. Eat three regular meals a day, breakfast and lunch kept small, with one main meal a day, either at lunchtime or in the evening. For the retired age group, the main meal should preferably be at mid-day.

Your diet for psychological illness should be naturally high in vitamins and minerals. Ideal foods are wholemeal bread, wheatgerm, vegetables, pulses, salads, and fish. Red meat should be avoided or kept low, with dairy products in moderation. Coffee, tea, and cocoa, should be avoided. They are acidic and their caffeine content is undesirable, briefly stimulating the nervous system, but leaving you feeling exhausted and low afterwards. It is also undesirable to encourage social addiction habits, as most tea or coffee drinking is a habit or part of a compulsive pattern. To avoid fluid retention, keep your intake of fluids moderate, except in the height of the summer or when there are very high humidity levels. Also avoid excessive amounts of salt or spices, as these tend to irritate the digestive and nervous system.

Avoid all forms of alcohol, until your psychological illness has been resolved and then enjoy it socially in moderation. Your diet should be high in vegetable fibre, preferably soluble fibre, which is found in oat bran. If possible obtain organic oat bran, as any pesticide residues are concentrated in the bran layer (to protect the wheatgerm) and levels are usually lower in organic products. Some fat is required, preferably as olive oil, but avoid fatty meals and fatty meat. Use raw, unrefined, sugar and wholemeal flour for cooking and baking. Minimise all snacks between meals, but particularly avoid chocolate, cakes, and high calorie foods such as nuts and crisps.

What you eat is important, but how you eat it also matters. Your food reflects your attitudes towards yourself, and this is often a major factor in recovery and health. As you become more healthy in your thinking and attitudes, you can also start to value yourself more, no longer taking your body for granted, or treating it as if it was unimportant, at times like a dustbin. Giving out more love and care, is also reflected in your overall concerns, and awareness, and this includes the quality of the food you give yourself. Stop eating instant or cheap, poor quality foods, and start repairing your body as well as your mind.

How you cook and prepare your food also matters. Lightly steam vegetables until they are just crisp, still firm, but not soggy. In this way, you will retain most of the vitamin content. Always grill, rather than fry, and reduce your intake of dishes which require a prolonged period of cooking, or heating to very high temperatures. Aim to eat lightly and as fresh as possible, with minimal intervention by the cooking process.

Avoid all supplements, during a psychological illness, unless they are recommended by your doctor. A daily vitamin or mineral pill, taken over a prolonged period of months or years, may eventually cause side-effects and undermine your health rather than promoting it.

Try to be sensible and balanced in what you eat and avoid being pernickety and obsessional. If you are depressed and have lost your appetite, eat little and often, but don't only eat out of a tin and try to concentrate on making a small meal attractive and presentable, as well as nutritious. As you come out of depression, you will naturally tend to eat more, but always keep to the same sensible principles of well-balanced meals which are fresh and nutritious.

DRUG-RELATED ILLNESS

Either prescribed or illicit drugs may be taken to excess and create psychological illness. Prescribed drugs, which are designed to alter the state of mind, are particularly problematic, especially for the elderly, but the younger age group may also be affected. Some drugs also undermine confidence or provoke anxiety attacks, at times causing problems of depression, dependency and panic.

Confusional states are common in the older age group, often the result of prescribed antidepressant or sedative drugs, which aim to relax the patient. They are usually given to help sleep problems, pain or allergy, but often provoke problems of nausea, agitation or confusion, as they tend to be only slowly excreted by the bowel or kidney, and in this way accumulate in the body, especially in the cells of the brain and nervous system. The patient may feel exhausted and tired, or there is an effect on judgement and fine co-ordinated movements, causing accident proneness, especially when taken with even small amounts of alcohol. Impotence and weakness are other common problems, especially following use of the circulatory beta-blocker type.

After taking antibiotics, many feel ill, depressed, and without energy. Some take months or years to recover their former drive and enthusiasm, as a result of the side-effects. Others develop chronic fungal infections, such as thrush.

Drugs of abuse, especially LSD, speed (amphetamines), Ecstasy, or Heroin, frequently cause confusional states, particularly if mixed as a cocktail with alcohol,

61

antidepressants, or tranquillisers, which can be very dangerous. Suicide is common, or violent attacks on others. A psychosis may occur. Many anti-depressant and anti-psychotic drugs cause tension, rigidity or tremor of the muscles and these effects may persist for months or years after the drug has been stopped.

Character traits which aggravate the condition
A tendency to dependant relationships and social addictions - tea, coffee, alcohol. Psychologically, he may rely too much on an older or younger sibling, husband or wife, who is allowed to take over decision-making, and in this way, weakens confidence and assertiveness.

Practical steps to improve things
If you are feeling unwell, lacking in confidence, unsure of yourself, after taking a particular drug, especially one for a psychological condition, always discuss this with your doctor to have his opinion on any possible connection with drugs taken. Your homoeopathic doctor may be able to order a specific antidote to the problem, as long as you can give details of the drug you were taking at the time. Avoid alcohol, coffee, tea, and cocoa, all of which act as stimulants and may lead to a low of energy, after any initial positive response. Keep yourself as fit as your health and age will allow. Exercise daily in the fresh air, walking is ideal. Eat a diet high in raw foods to encourage elimination. Try to clarify why you first needed to start taking drugs, for example, an underlying problem of depression, and the feelings which led you to become dependent upon a chemical 'prop', which may have originally been either prescribed or taken illegally.

Remedies to consider:-

Camphor

A remedy for states of exhaustion, the body cold and empty of all energy. At other times, the mind is excited, fearful, in a state of anguish. He has impulses to attack or destroy others, talking irrationally. Depressed and irritable, there may be high levels of anxiety, often a conviction that he is condemned or evil, fears usually worse at night when he feels guilt-ridden and bad. He cannot tolerate being covered in bed. There is a tendency for small spasmodic movements to occur, spasms or tics. At times he seems on the brink of a coma.

Cannabis indica

There is an excitable state of mind, the thoughts incoherent, with vague, speculative ideas, e.g. does he exist, for what purpose, is he about to die? At other times, he is depressed or despairing. Hallucinations are heard or seen, especially evil figures, demons, or he hears music and singing. He is convinced he has a double. Many of the thoughts are omnipotent and dangerous, for example, that he can fly. Time is distorted, and passes very slowly. A few minutes may seem like centuries. The body size is distorted in terms of length, distance and shape. Moods vary from laughter to depression. Overall he is absent-minded, unable to concentrate, full of ideas which take over the mind. Memory and concentration are poor.

Natrum mur

Indicated for tall, thin, exhausted constitutions. There is an irritable, silent indifferent state of mind, depressed and weeping, quickly becoming irritable. He prefers to be alone, is worse for reassurance or consolation and is rigid and hypochondriacal. Intolerant of criticism, clumsy, hesitant, he finds concentration difficult because of chronic fatigue. He is never at ease in any social situation. Salt is craved, and fluid retention causes discomfort.

Opium

For an irritable, over-talkative, confused state of mind. The face is red and congested, eyes glistening. He is fearful and apprehensive, seeing visions of animals, or approaching death. At times he is sullen, weak, depressed, dull and apathetic, unable to concentrate and has an overwhelming desire to sleep. He may become withdrawn, insensible, the breathing loud and snoring, not responding to pain or any stimulus. Constipation is often a severe problem. There may be a tremor of the head, sudden muscular jerking, or tics of the limbs. He is hypersensitive to noise, bright lights and odours.

Sulphur

Indicated for an agitated state of mind, with morbid guilt-ridden ideas, that he has neglected his job or business. He may talk in a vague speculative, philosophical way, full of arrogant pride, or idealises old clothes and rags as beautiful. Memory is poor, and at times he can be spiteful or irritable. There is an absence of enjoyment. Burning pains, of the rectum, bladder, stomach, intestine, uterus are common. Due to circulation problems, the face and head are hot and red, the hands and feet ice cold. He dislikes washing, and is worse for heat. Chronic skin problems are a feature, often infected and discharging pus. On waking, an offensive diarrhoea usually drives him from the bed.

DRUG WITHDRAWAL

Stopping any drug, once dependency has occurred, may lead to the most devastating physical symptoms. These include nausea, constipation, tremor, feeling faint or cold, problems of fear, panic, tension or agitation, and lack of confidence. Much publicity has been given in the past to the problems addicts face when trying to come off Heroin or other opium-based drugs. The 'cold turkey' state of the depressed addict, although now helped by substitute drugs such as Methadone, can still be a lonely state of indescribable agony.

It is only in recent years, that doctors have come to realise that trying to control the dependency problems which develop after taking certain prescribed tranquillisers, can be just as difficult and devastating.

The process of coming off prescribed anti-depressant or tranquilliser drugs taken over a long period, may take months or years. This still poses a major problem for many patients, who although now symptom-free, lack the will and the confidence to stop their drugs because they fear a relapse or a panic attack, as soon as they stop or reduce their dosage. There is a tendency to perpetuate the dependency and insecurity feelings by carrying a reserve supply of pills - 'for use in an emergency'. Any mild digestive complaint, infection, or flu, can cause a sensation of feeling hot and faint, weak in the stomach area. The drugs may again be taken as a reaction of panic, the patient further drawn into dependency, each new symptom re-enforcing the habit.

Character traits which aggravate the condition

The main problem is often pessimism, fear of becoming ill again, having another breakdown. There is a lack of confidence, a tendency to panic at minor symptoms of anxiety, to feel vulnerable, taken over by depression, fear, lack of control and feelings of acute agitation.

Practical steps to improve things

Try to relax more, not only when you are tense, but throughout the day, but especially when you are with others, driving the car, in the theatre, or at any time when anxiety takes over your peace of mind.

If you are trying to come off any drug of addiction, you will probably require some help and support. You will almost certainly need to find a trusted friend or professional worker, who you can talk to and who will help you resolve the many different emotions which emerge as you stop taking the drug and break the dependency habit. Try to work at all areas of your dependency, and aim to be less passive or dependant when you are with others and more assertive and definite in your arguments and opinions. Don't agree or disagree, for the sake of it. Remain in close contact with your essential individuality in all things, not allowing yourself to be dominated or taken over by old resentments, familiar patterns, workaholic routines or hard-line attitudes. Try to listen and be more flexible, developing new friendships, exploring new pathways of interest, enjoyment and self-expression.

Remedies to consider:-

Argentum nit   There is a state of impatient mental agitation, with marked phobic anxiety, panic attacks, apathy or exhaustion. A marked tremor occurs because of high levels of tension. There is often a mood of silent depression, and hypochondriacal fears are common. Sharp, stitch-like pains may occur in any part of the body. Time seems to pass slowly, and all symptoms are worse from heat.

Natrum mur   A remedy for drug withdrawal problems, when there is a state of exhaustion and tearful depression. He is usually tall, thin, clumsy and irritable, preferring solitude to company, but needing a great deal of reassurance. There is a confused state of mind, with dizziness. Salt is craved and all symptoms are worse for sea air.

Nux vomica   For short-fuse irritability of mood and impulses to violence, to break or destroy objects. He is over-sensitive to cold air, noise, bright light or odours. Silent, morose, often fearful, hypochondriacal, he is nearly always over-zealous or too intense. Time passes too slowly. He is rarely satisfied, complaining, negative, agitated and pessimistic. Concentration and memory are poor, and the bowels are usually constipated. There may be a tendency to suicide or homicide.

Opium A remedy for confused, excitable, irritable moods, with a tendency to deliberately mislead or deceive. A state of delirium may develop. The face is red, the eyes open and glistening. He is imaginative and fearful, with visions of phantoms or ghosts which persecute him. At other times he is in an apathetic, tired, intoxicated state of mind, insensitive to any form of stimulation or pain. The head feels dizzy. He may become comatose, with heavy, snoring breathing, or many sudden tremors or fluttering movements. Constipation is usually a severe problem. There is dislike of bright light, noise or odour.

The specific drug involved, taken in homoeopathic potency.

FEAR STATES

There is an overwhelming feeling of tension, anxiety and panic, particularly when a demand or change is required. Usually a specific event causes apprehension and uncertainty, often because it is new and unfamiliar. Symptoms of apprehension may be present for months before an anticipated event actually occurs. The major source of fear is often leaving a known position of relative security. This varies from:- changing school, moving house or employment, an interview, examination, or assessment. Even leaving home to go on holiday or a visit, may cause fear to intensify, if security levels are low, or there are phobic problems. Fear is typically associated with feeling open and exposed to failure or criticism, in some way at risk, without support or adequate defense against laughter or ridicule. Such anxieties are more about fear than any reality rejection and usually relate to infantile insecurity problems, anxiety about lack of support or understanding, but especially loss of love and affection by the parents and terror of their anger or rejection.

Fear may have been triggered by a specific incident, perhaps an accident, or a near-death experience, on the road, in a plane, when playing as a child, or something quite banal may have happened, such as a painful fall. Often the cause dates to an overwhelming reaction by the parents to a relatively minor childhood incident. Typical examples include:- when an exploring and rather independent toddler gets lost in the woods. Also falling off a child's bicycle seat onto the road (just as a lorry was passing), or perhaps seeing it happen to another toddler and sensing the panic and reaction of the parents, especially if they always tended to over-react to every emotional situation, in this way provoking the child's first experience of terror and insecurity.

Fear is often engendered by these excessive reactions (panic, anger, hysteria) of the adult(s) present at the time, rather than what actually happened in the child's own mind. The root of fear may also have occurred at school, associated with teasing and bullying (or fear of it) by other children or a particular teacher. Others may have been made to feel different, picked upon, given a denigrating name or label, not invited to join the playground 'gang', to play games with the other children. In some cases the child was simply ignored because he was fat, shy, intellectual, odd, or culturally different from the other children. Sometimes bullying or abuse of an older sibling was observed, but never talked about. Most children have experienced at least one trauma or severe fright at some time in their life, but it did not lead to a sense of overwhelming fear, because it was handled with calm understanding, patience and sensitivity at the time.

Character traits which aggravate the condition

There is a tendency to be over-imaginative, to anticipate failure or difficulties, always pessimistic, rather than positive or forward-looking in attitudes. The underlying emotions are depressive and negative, often looking for proof of rejection and failure, rather than seeing each new occasion as a challenge and a possibility for greater self-expression.

Practical steps to improve things

Aim to explore any new and frightening situation, in order to learn more about yourself and your attitudes to moving outside narrow and usually familiar boundaries and experiences. Treat each state of fear as a possible key to change and as an area you need to know more about. Specific areas of fear can be usefully considered as a front-line action area, for growth and change. This may involve:- meeting others, going out to new and unfamiliar situations, shopping, or driving on a motorway or moving further away from the security of your home base. The origins of this kind of problem usually occurred in infancy, and the attitudes have often been there since childhood. See the problem as relating to an infantile part of yourself, which tries to dominate you with its fears and attitudes. Try talking to this part of you, getting to know and making friends with it, trying to engender trust at this level, before going into a new or potential fear situation. Before any new threatening situation, talk to this infantile part of you, to contact and reassure it, but always explaining what the realities are and if possible try to understand why this infantile part of you is over-sensitive and sees change as such a threat. Work at this area slowly, in a positive loving way, exactly as if caring for a small frightened child.

Remedies to consider:-

Aconitum

A remedy for acute violent states of fear, marked by restless agitation. The mood is irritable and variable. There is fear of death, ghosts, the dark or any new unfamiliar situation. Depressed, weeping, moaning, agitated moods may occur, which cannot be easily consoled. Music aggravates all the symptoms.

Arsenicum

For obsessional fears, with burning pains and weakness. He feels cold and chilly, even at the height of summer, wearing several layers of clothes. Heat is craved throughout the year.

Aurum met

Indicated for tearful moods of despondency, anguish and fear. There is a sense of hopelessness, often a compulsive determination to acts of self-destruction and suicide. He feels guilty, hopeless, despairing, often complaining of palpitations and rheumatic joint pains. He is hyper-sensitive to cold air, touch, and at the same time, intolerant and quick to anger with moods of irritability.

73

Argentum nit There is apathy with restlessness and hypochondriacal fears. He is silent, withdrawn, fearing failure, leaving home or travelling. The memory is poor. Bizarre thoughts trouble him and undermine confidence. Flatulence is a common problem, often feeling full and bloated and usually worse from heat.

Belladonna For variable fears, the face red, pulse rapid, pupils dilated. He is intolerant of draughts of air, light, noise or touch. Confusion may occur, becoming acutely psychotic and hallucinated, terrified of the dark, insects and 'things' in his room. At times he can become violent or spiteful, with impulses to bite.

Borax There is nervous agitation, related to any form of forward or downward movement, for example, in an aeroplane, going downstairs, an escalator, rocking chair, or when leaning forward. He has no drive or interest in work.

Calcarea For a fair but flabby constitution, with a tendency to sweat on the head area. He is always cold, often despondent, with variable moods of fear and anxiety, accompanied by palpitations and vertigo. He fears 'something'will happen, particularly fearful of death or the dark. Slow and exhausted, concentration is poor and worse after any intellectual effort. There are many obsessional features in his thinking.

Calcarea phos

Indicated for a tall, thin, dark complexioned person, who is full of gloomy fearful thoughts, often associated with recurrent headaches. Anguish is felt in the pit of the stomach. Levels of concentration are poor and he is quickly irritable.

Cicuta

For states of anguish with mood changes. Fears cause a sinking sensation in the chest region. Everything seems strange, dangerous, or terrifying, and suspicion is marked. He prefers to be alone, often tearful, depressed, tense with many tics and odd mannerisms due to tension or an excitable state of mind. He is startled by the least sound, quick to anger or violence.

Digitalis   A remedy for mixed states of depression and fear. There is anxiety about illness and dying, with lack of confidence. He is pessimistic and irritable, often indifferent in mood, wanting to withdraw from life or any new challenge. Palpitations are a source of anxiety. A state of apathy prevails.

Gelsemium   For hysterical states of fear, with terror of appearing in public, also examinations, interviews, or any situation where he feels he may be critically assessed.

Graphites   For states of apprehension and fear, weeping depression, and anxiety. He prefers to be alone, timid and hesitant, but is easily irritable, weighed down by life's 'problems' reflecting feelings of inadequacy. Skin eruptions are common, typically moist and with a clear or yellowish discharge.

Hydrophobinum   A remedy for fear of madness, all symptoms aggravated by the thought or sight of water or any liquid. Convulsions, fits, spasm, tics, odd mannerisms and gesticulations are common, relating to the underlying tension, and the anxiety.

Ignatia

There is a weeping depression, with confused feelings of fear and timidity. He is full of guilt and self-reproach, quickly irritated, moody and fearful of intruders, illness, especially cancer. All symptoms are related to a recent loss, disappointment or anniversary reaction. He feels disappointed, let down, angry, and these feelings tend to become obsessional, dominating all other forms of thinking and ideas. There is a feeling of weakness, particularly in the stomach area.

Kali arsen

Indicated for restless, nervous states of behaviour, with depression. Intolerable skin itching is a common feature. Any infected areas, tend to discharge pus.

Lycopodium

A remedy for anticipatory fears, and problems of immaturity. Everything is rushed, done in a hurry, with a 'butterfly' mind, which is distracted and inattentive, constantly seeking reassurance. Ill-timed, quick movements lead to accident-proneness. All symptoms are worse in the early evening from 4-8.00 pm.

Natrum carb

Fair complexion, depressed and fearful. Weakness is a marked feature. Anxious and restless, lonely and irritable, he sweats profusely on the face and head. Fearful of noise and bright lights, concentration is poor, all symptoms aggravated by heat or music, the latter causing a tearful mood of sadness.

Phosphorus

Indicated for a tall, often red-haired person, with tight chesty breathing problems. There are many problems of anxiety and fear. Apathy is marked. Depressed and sad, he dreads illness or the future, constantly seeking recognition and reassurance. Burning body pains are characteristic, and he is always chilly, yet craves ice-cold drinks. Exhaustion occurs after the least physical or mental effort.

Platinum

For egotistical, haughty, proud states of mind, with an exaggerated sense of his self-importance. Fears and mood changes are marked. He is reserved and cold, seeing others as small or inferior. Tension causes tight, band-like headaches or limb pains.

Psorinum

There is an anxious fearful state of mind, constantly weeping and fearing death, or a business failure. Palpitations are frequent, with chest oppression and a sense of anguish. There are major mood changes. Self-willed, obstinate, and irritable, he has a low motivation for work, and both memory and concentration are poor. There is often an accompanying skin infection, with deep infected cracks, the skin grey and dirty-looking.

Sepia

The personality is negative, defeatist, cold and irritable. He is always worse for music, but feels better from dancing or vigorous exercise. Depression causes apathy, tiredness, a feeling of being worn out or dragged down by fatigue and worrying about his health and life's problems. Low back pain is a chronic problem. He is often bored or indifferent to to everyone, over-sensitive to noise, odour, bright lights, and social contacts. There is a characteristic brown saddle-shaped marking on the bridge of the nose.

Stramonium For excitable states of fear, with violent outbursts, confused, deluded, biting and scratching. He is convinced there is an immediate threat to his life, fearful of being attacked and often anxious when left alone in a room. He is hallucinated, seeing insects or animals in the room. There is an aversion to water and liquids. All movements are quick and clumsy. The body image is distorted, one limb, or sometimes the whole body feels too tall or enlarged. Moods vary from laughter to screaming rage, dancing, singing, swearing or fighting. All symptoms are worse after sleep.

HALLUCINATIONS

These are essentially a projection of the inner workings of the mind onto everyday reality happenings. Fleeting hallucinations may occur from physical causes, especially a high temperature, drug abuse, alcohol, and states of severe malnutrition. But on the whole, these are the rare exceptions, the cause usually obvious. In most cases, there is an underlying psychological illness, with a break with reality leading to misperception and hallucinations.

Hallucinations may be seen, heard, felt, or sometimes they occur as a faint but persistent odour. Most common are the auditory distortions with fragments of the mind felt to taunt and provoke the individual with threats and provocations, sometimes of an overt sexual nature. Others occur as 'visions', or a sense of being watched, touched or prodded.

Every hallucination reflects the energy from an isolated, fragmented thought or feeling, revolving within a delusional psychotic state of mind and not fully integrated into any picture of overall reality. The patient fails to differentiate between his inner world of dreams and omnipotent fantasies, and an outer more mundane, at times powerless or tedious, often impotent world of difficulty, compromise, negotiation, relationships and reality. The hallucinations tend to recall and repeat the same theme, over and over again, in a distorted often rigid way which limits self-expression. This may be related to a past hurt or rejection, what was said, or at times not said, but imagined. Psychologically, all growth of a vulnerable, sensitive part of the self, is blocked or fixated, 'stuck in a groove' like an old 78

81

record echoing the same feeling over and over again. This preoccupation with a particular hurt or provocation, makes it difficult to change or come to terms with it. Progress may be slow or blocked because there is fear of a further rejection, because feelings and needs are strong, or it is feared that reactions of anger or flight may occur and make the situation worse.

Case report
One young adult became preoccupied with sexual thoughts. She felt unattractive, that she lacked sexual appeal and feared being raped, if she became involved or attracted to a man. Her psychotic illness caused frequent auditory hallucinations repeating 'Your mind has been raped'. Visual hallucinations also occurred, seeing faces with a long pointed nose (probably a phallic symbol). She still felt aggrieved, concerning a college student, who had made provocative sexual remarks to her in the past, and then failed to ask her out or made any attempt at a relationship. She felt a mixture of anger and hurt, often fearful and aroused, frequently rejected and humiliated.

The problem was aggravated by the apparent success of her sister, the fact that she had a regular boy-friend, and was popular, and she felt intensely irritated by her laughter. The combination of festering emotions, with frustrated unexpressed sexual emotions, (really libidinal energy), became destructive, and led to a severe psychotic breakdown with a prolonged period of delusional illness, at times suicidal in intensity. As a result of homoeopathy, the hallucinations subsided, and there was a marked diminution of the psychotic illness.

Often the causes of a psychotic illness are less clear, and hallucinations are the first manifestation of a more insidious process, undermining rational thinking and relationships.

Sometimes hallucinations become more threatening, especially in a paranoid (persecutory) illness. They may develop an omnipotent grandiose element, to save the world, chosen by God for a special mission, in order to compensate for underlying feelings of inferiority and inadequacy.

Character traits which aggravate the condition
The previous personality is often shy, sensitive, withdrawn and socially isolated. There is a tendency to day-dream and take flight from reality challenges and personal problems into fantasy or mystical theoretical ideas. Self-trust is often low and others are kept at a distance, increasingly living in a world of secrecy and mystery.

Practical steps to improve things
The best approach by far is prevention, tackling at an early age, any attempt by a shy child to withdraw or retreat into a world of fantasy, as soon as it occurs. Of course, fantasy and imagination are healthy and normal for all children and occur naturally, as part of play. But the family should be aware of any tendency to be unduly quiet, withdrawn, depressed, or passive, persisting in a fantasy world, rather than wanting to learn, explore and have contact with other children. If abnormal shyness or timidity occurs in an older child, this can be effectively treated homoeopathically. In adolescence, it can be treated by combining homoeopathy with the same open approach and

extended sensitive dialogue, which should involve the whole family. Counselling or deeper more intensive psychotherapeutic help may be required.

If you are an adult and experiencing hallucinations, try not to allow them to totally dominate you or to take over. Maintain contacts with others, and talk about any 'voices or visions' you are experiencing with a trusted friend, or in any treatment group situation you may be attending. If you don't feel you can trust anyone sufficiently to be able to discuss this, then try to see the 'voices' as reflecting a part of you which has become detached, and then developed an energy and direction of its own. Try also to understand that every hallucination, each experience of a voice or vision is really an attempt by an isolated part of you to become re-integrated (or whole) within you. To that extent it is a positive experience and one you can support, as long as you don't allow this fragmented part of your mind to overwhelm your totality. Aim to recall and understand any traumatic early childhood experiences, which may have led to a splitting off of powerful feelings and emotions within your mind.

Remedies to consider:-

Belladonna

There is an irritable restless state of anger, often fury, with a tendency to bite. The face is typically red, the hallucinations accompanied by vertigo and confusion of mind. Visual hallucinations of dogs, wolves, mice, insects, seem to swarm over the table or up the walls. He also sees ghosts, giants, or fire. A state of terror may occur.

Cannabis ind

A remedy for hallucinations which are fantastic and distorted. They may occur in colour, the body transparent, enlarged or distorted, sparks flying off him. Elation may give the sensation of being on horseback.

Hyoscyamus

For excitable states of mind, restless and talkative, deluded or confused. There is a tendency to tear off his clothes, or become violent. Moods vary from one moment to another. Visual and auditory hallucinations occur, with withdrawal from others, muttering or chattering away about delusional beliefs and cut off from reality within a psychotic fantasy world.

Stramonium   Violent outbursts are often due to visual hallucinations of insects, dogs, or rabbits, felt to be all around the room. There is fear of water, and dislike of all forms of liquid, also of the dark. Moods vary from one extreme to another.

Sulphur   Recommended for more long-term chronic problems. There is a marked distortion and idealisation of everyday objects. Even old rags are seen as beautiful, an old hat or coat, felt to be attractive and desirable. There are many religious or speculative philosophical ideas, moods varying from anxiety to a weeping depression, at times agitated or irritable. He tends to be untidy, neglected and dirty looking. All the mental symptoms are worse from heat.

HYSTERIA

A hysterical illness is always marked by a strong sense
of the dramatic, placing the person into the limelight, as
much as he protests that it is the last thing wanted. The
symptoms are variable, often frightening and they
typically cause alarm or sympathy, in the doctor, friends
and family. Hysteria closely mimics the most serious of
conditions, often defying either diagnosis or cure.
Usually the patient suddenly improves from a
complicated illness, with an inexplicable or spontaneous
cure, that leaves you feeling helpless or terrified.
Typically the hysteric is desperate, lying in a faint, pale
as marble, the cheeks or lips purple and seemingly at
death's door. At other times, he is involved in
threatening emotional situations. There may have been
dramatic emotional scenes, which rival any media
'soap' with floods of tears and laughter, scenes of
passion, hate, jealousy, violence, timidity, threats, but at
other times delicate and caring. The extremes of
emotion vary from one crisis to another.

The hysteric is never fully relaxed or natural with other
adults, always tense and on guard, slightly embarrassed
and shy, at the same time, inevitably drawing attention
to himself. He is usually very popular with children,
and naturally able to reach down to their level, and can
mimic or play effectively, just like a small child, at the
same time enjoying the attention this brings. It is never
possible to be certain of his mood, except to say that it
will be dramatic, unpredictable and usually exhausting.

Character traits which aggravate the condition

There is a childish aspect to the personality, always seeking reassurance, threatened by aging and fearful of death. Youth and appearance are far too important and this is why each birthday is a major tragedy and a threat. Insecurity is marked, and like a child, they gather parental or authority figures around them who they win over or seduce in one way or another; at the same time creating problems of jealousy and rivalry. The whole of life may be ruled by a series of dramas and intrigues, either real or imagined. They are excellent in the theatre, or in any situation where lively drama and appearance is important.

Practical steps to improve things

Aim to increase the depth of your relationships, at the same time, becoming more aware of any childish aspects of your behaviour. Try to link these up with your actual early experiences, to understand how your present dramas and problems are a continuation of this much earlier way of coping with others, and your overall development. Develop new relationships with all age groups, and a wide varied group of people, working on the relationships to keep them open, spontaneous and caring. Aim to see how you import the same kind of dramatic infantile themes into all your relationships and that these are destructive and often leave you isolated and frustrated. Clarify the patterns in your life and how they are repeated. It often helps to discuss this with a close friend, and try not to take too seriously any dramas which come up. Aim to understand the reasons for these patterns of behaviour and the links with your early developmental experiences in childhood.

Remedies to consider:-

Argentum nit For hysterical states with marked phobic obsessional fears and often a lump in the throat. There is intolerance of heat.

Asafoetida Indicated for mild hysterical anxiety states, fainting easily, with chronic indigestion problems and flatulence.

Gelsemium A remedy for wild states of apprehension, lack of confidence, feeling especially vulnerable and exposed when appearing in a public situation.

Lycopodium For anticipatory hysterical fears with agitation, always crossing bridges before they occur. He tends to rush ahead in all matters, taking risks, too intense, fearing disapproval and always needing to be popular and liked.

Pulsatilla Change and variability of mood, drive and direction are the main psychological characteristics of this remedy. Moods vary from irritation and anger, to tears or uncontrollable laughter, but always excessive, dramatic or posed. There is intolerance of heat and lack of thirst.

INDECENT EXPOSURE

Indecent exposure is not strictly a psychological illness, and can be regarded as more of a social or relationship problem. The act usually denies underlying feelings of desperation, futility, often severe tension or depression, and for this reason I have decided to include it. It is also a very common stress problem. It is nearly always a male sexual problem, reflecting nervousness, insecurity and immaturity, associated with fear as well as distortion of women.

The act of provoking the female by briefly exposing the erect penis, keeps him at a safe distance and one where he is in control and can control the viewing. There is flight from feared dependency needs, and a close mature relationship. Chronic depression is a common underlying feature. The man may be married, but unhappy or emotionally isolated from his wife and children. Another cause may be a particularly severe period of stress, which has not been shared and talked through. More rarely the cause is a psychotic delusional illness, usually of a schizophrenic type.

Sometimes the man concerned has failed to ever achieve a fully committed closeness to any woman and has developed a series of distant relationships which never allowed trust, dependency or loving closeness to develop. He may be highly successful at work, or in sport, but has a compulsion to expose himself in order to obtain sexual satisfaction. Usually the act relates to infantile impulses, dating back to a time in his life when he was damaged psychologically, and failed to fully mature. The overwhelming need is to briefly experience power over women (symbolically a dominating mother).

The act of exposure may reassure him briefly but quickly leads to guilt feelings and frustration.

If the exposure becomes compulsive it may also undermine professional work and concentration, at times creating a physical risk.

Case report
One man in his early 30's, with this type of problem, only exposed himself when in a car, driving at speed. He would regularly expose himself briefly when overtaking a coach containing female passengers, and at this time was a danger to himself and to other road users. He was alienated from his wife and children, but very successful professionally. The key issue was a very unhappy early childhood relationship, with a dominating mother and a weak distant father, who failed to act as a buffer to the mother, or become a figure he could respect and identify with.

The kind of problem usually has its roots in childhood, in a complex psychological process. There is usually lack of confidence with women and a restricted upbringing which caused his sexuality to become repressed, i.e. denied, or pushed down, linked to guilt, shame and rigid attitudes. Psychologically, he may have been an only child, or had much older siblings with insufficient social contact with a sister or female companions during his formative years.

Character traits which aggravate the condition

Insecurity is marked towards the opposite sex, with remoteness, particularly within a marriage or existing relationship. There is a tendency to keep stress pressures locked within, especially feelings of anger, anxiety or insecurity. These are not usually talked about or shown. Immaturity is a feature, especially when under pressure, with feelings out of control. This may lead to repetitive childish, attention-seeking behaviour in many areas of life. There is a strong wish to be looked at and reassured, seeking acceptance and approval from a distance and always fearing a close affectionate relationship.

Practical steps to improve things

Try to break with old infantile ways of hiding emotions and needs by more direct open sharing of yourself with others. Aim to be more of an individual, spontaneous and giving, not just problems and fears, but more fundamental feelings, such as joy, sadness or laughter. Sexual needs and fantasies should be openly talked about with your partner, discussing intimate feelings as part of your closeness and a sharing relationship. Try also to be more open with feelings of affection, less shut away and remote. If you are not in a relationship, in the middle of a divorce, a major stress situation, try to make new friends, both male and female, and develop new areas of interest with them. If the problem persists, in addition to basic homoeopathy, consider a period of counselling or therapy, but discuss this first with your homoeopathic doctor.

Remedies to consider:-

Gelsemium   Fear and lack of confidence are the main causes of the problem. Dizziness with weakness is a common problem area. Sexual drive and potency is weak.

Natrum mur   The exposure problem is usually a reaction to an underlying depressive problem, with needs to gain attention, yet fearing any close or real contact with others.

Pulsatilla   The temperament is variable and dramatic, often depressed or tearful. With the exception of masturbation, there is a total lack of confidence in any direct sexual situation, yet a constant need to gain attention.

Silicea   Weakness is marked with loss of drive. He is often underweight, always cold, covered with sweat and usually lacking confidence. There is fear of close contact with women. A fixed compulsive behaviour pattern causes the act to be repeated.

MANIC-DEPRESSIVE PSYCHOSIS

This is a major illness, marked by severe mood swings, periods of extreme excitement and overactivity, alternating with periods of profound depression and despair. There are many psychological and chemical theories about the illness, and much research has been carried out, but the cause still remains unknown.

In a manic or 'high' phase of the illness, drive is boundless, also enthusiasm and energy. The mind is optimistic and eager, full of plans, ideas, optimism, energy and drive. At times the mind seems to accelerate headlong, leaping from one idea to another. There is a tendency to over-work, waking early, talking, planning, arranging meetings or projects into the early hours, brimming over with exciting ideas, sometimes filling books or scraps of paper, with thoughts and associations which crowd into the mind. Eventually a delusional state develops with no insight into the excesses. Risks may be taken with family or personal savings, often spending or gambling thousands, leaving essential bills neglected, spending hours on the telephone, confiding and indiscreet. At other times suspicion of friends or the family comes to the fore, with a conviction that those close are 'plotting' to have him locked away, or there is an international spy ring or political scandal, which he knows about and is about to disclose. Name-dropping of royalty, political or world leaders, is common. Success at business and a high level of intelligence can make many elements of the grandiose (delusional) plots seem plausible. Mistrust and suspicions may make it difficult to call a doctor or a psychiatrist, because any period of observation or treatment, is seen as a form of deliberate and plotted infringement of liberty. During the manic phase, the characteristic delusional element of a psychotic illness is never far away, and from time to time it takes over, in a very persuasive way, with a conviction beyond any doubt of the correctness of his beliefs and assertions.

A depressive phase inevitably follows the 'high' of the manic period. There is a reversal of the drive, energy levels and buoyant optimism. The patient sinks into a deep pit of despair and fatigue, needing to sleep, get away, not wanting to wake up, avoiding others, or face up to the problems and 'mess' he feels he has created. But even in the midst of the self-recriminations, the delusional grandiose element is still present. The problems and disasters caused are earth-shattering, everyone knows about them, are talking about him. The 'havoc' he has caused is beyond repair and forgiveness. Feelings are often intensely self-destructive. Relaxation and rest may at times become impossible because of the intensity of guilt feelings, a sense of complete and utter failure and feeling worthless.

Despair and lack of drive, makes him convinced he is a nuisance, unloved by all, a liability to friends and family, and that the sooner he is dead, the better for all. Suicidal thoughts may become obsessional, constantly on his mind, when and how, planned silently but deliberately, and felt to be the only option left open to him.

Case Study

A young man with a manic-depressive psychotic illness, came home on weekend leave from a psychiatric hospital. He appeared to have improved over the past weeks, and came to attend a family wedding. He seemed to enjoy himself, chatting to friends and family, appearing relaxed and happy. The family confidently left him alone for a short time in the late afternoon. During that period he tragically threw himself from a high building.

Character traits which aggravate the condition

There is a tendency to be volatile in all emotional responses, to get overwhelmed with the pressure and pace of everyday things, rushing and tense, usually because you are not sufficiently relaxed and taking things slowly. You tend to become far too pressurised and wound-up by events, instead of taking them more slowly and step by step.

Practical steps to improve things

Try to stay relaxed during the day, with regular rest breaks. Forget the pressures, and give yourself more time to clear the mind. Aim to be less intense in your approach to stress and anxiety, pacing yourself, when under pressure. If there is a problem, either at work or in the home, try not to take the whole burden on your shoulders, but share it more with colleagues, your spouse, or partner. Delegate more, and if you feel tensions building up, becoming restless, unable to sleep, or still in top gear late in the evening, then take a few hours off to ease the pressures. Try getting away from any family, social, or stress situations, forgetting about work and tensions.

Remedies to consider:-

Aconitum

The face is bright red due to the excitable mood state. There are rapid changes of emotion, with confusion, irritability, impatience, and restlessness. Everything is done in a hurry. Fear is always present, going out, the dark, of imminent death. Depression is a problem, with obstinate and apprehensive attitudes to others, all symptoms worse from music and cold air.

Belladonna

The head is congested, the face hot, dark or purple pink, the eyes staring, pupils dilated. There is a confused state of mind, restless, and excitable, with visions and hallucinations. Irritability can quickly turn to rage or fury. At other times, the mood is one of weeping despair, full of anguish, suspicion, and mistrust. He is convinced that death is imminent. There is extreme hyper-sensitivity to noise, cold air, touch. Sudden spasms of pain occur in the throat, stomach, rectum, bladder or uterus.

Hyoscyamus

This remedy is indicated for extremely excitable confused manic states of mind. Delusional beliefs drive the patient from his bed, often into violent moods. At times he makes inappropriate gestures, holds unreasonable beliefs, is depressed and tearful, or moved to laughter. Typical depressive delusions are a conviction that he is already dead, and has been devoured by animals. There is a marked aversion to any form of liquid, especially water. Concentration is weak, and he quickly loses his train of thought. Vertigo is common, also muscular spasms, tics, fits, contractions.

Natrum mur

The patient is usually thin, tall, chilly and weak, often bowed over with a tearful depression. Irritable, at times indifferent, he is often haughty and distant, always worse for consolation or reassurance. At other times he can suddenly switch moods, and become excited, singing and laughing. Much of the time he is hypochondriacal and fearful, seeking to be alone, apathetic and distant. The illness often occurs following an emotional shock, disappointment, or rejection.

Stramonium

A remedy for violent often uncontrollable manic states. He is deluded, fearful of the dark, being attacked by dogs, convinced that death is imminent. Overwhelmed by anxiety, he sees an array of animals running around the room, or horrible beasts which threaten to destroy him. Devils or threatening faces torment and tease him. He has a strong aversion to all fluids. Even the thought of them can cause an irritable spasm of the pharynx (throat). The fingers are restless, picking at the covers, or small imagined objects on the floor. He experiences murderous impulses to attack, bite, scratch others, based on fear.

Tarentula

A remedy for the most excitable restless states of mind. He acts in a destructive way, tearing at the bed clothes, striking out, scratching or cutting his wrists, pulling out his hair. The mental agitation is worse for music, bright colours and at night. Moods are changeable, singing, sad or dejected, tearful or moaning. Memory is poor.

MENTAL ILLNESS

Mental or mind illness can take many shapes and forms. A common problem is the need to control all emotions and spontaneity, leading to a personality which is apparently strong and independent, but in reality, rigid and unable to show feelings. Some patients are intolerant because they were never fully allowed to be a child, too quickly pushed into the adult role, and disapproved of when ill or showed any signs of vulnerability or weakness. In later life, any feelings, upset, or emotion, may be experienced as physical discomfort, developing a deep-seated abdominal pain, perhaps an irritable bowel problem, rather than showing tears. This type of upbringing, may lead to a tendency to become over-conforming, never taking a risk or a chance in life, in order to avoid the possibility of failure. This is because failure at anything has come to symbolise being rejected, alienated from the love, care and the respect of others. There may be a tendency to create rigid controlled attitudes, involving both the self and others, the result of a need for constant attention and reassurance, but essentially to stay in control and to be less vulnerable. Creativity, the capacity for a new more imaginative approach to life tends to be curtailed or absent, although there are exceptions, when an exceptional talent continues to reveal itself, despite the illness process. But in my experience this is quite rare. Symptoms vary from extreme periods of excitable gregarious activity, to low moods of fatigue, despair, and withdrawal from others. The psychological damage may cause a permanent flattening of mood leading to a bland 'normality', conforming, reliable, predictable but boring. The efficiency and regularity may give no clues to the underlying torment and depths of anxiety felt. A total obliteration of any emotional problems may occur, often denying that the feelings and emotions exist at all, as life is reduced to a predictable, efficient, machine-like, meaningless routine.

At other times, fear of confrontation and argument leads to refusal to discuss a strongly held point-of-view. Conflict, argument, or dispute of any kind, may be kept hidden, until persistent, odd, or inappropriate behaviour draws attention to the possibility of an underlying psychological illness. Stealth, obstinacy, cunning and manipulation of the family may be early manifestations of mental illness, often linked to a family where there is poor communication, lacking sympathy and a softer, more gentle, subtle approach to family tensions.

Depression and suicide are increasingly common in young people, as violence has come to be part of normal social expression. Rigid obsessional controls, with denial of need and vulnerability may eventually lead to a persecutory and delusional type of illness, or a senile confusional state in later years.

Despite many years of debate and research, the cause of many forms of mental illness is still not fully understood. There have been many arguments about possible physical causation, chemical or hormonal imbalance, lack of vitamins, viral or other infective agents, as well as theories advocating a psychological cause following a traumatic or unsatisfactory early experience in infancy or childhood leading to negative conditioning of the patient. The arguments still continue and inconsistent hormonal and biochemical levels are sometimes found, although it has never been proven whether they are cause or effect. It is quite likely that

101

any hormonal changes which occur, act as a trigger mechanism to release unstable (damaged) areas of the psyche, which in most cases are associated with a trauma or rejection occurring in the early formative years.

The main diagnostic pointers to mental illness are:-
a loss of judgement and insight into the condition and often alienation or withdrawal. Events and experiences are reacted to, rather than with, because they are felt to be part of a delusional process which is dominated by fantasy. People, gestures, remarks, suggestions, language, are all felt to confirm the delusional convictions. During the acute stage of the illness, it may be quite impossible to modify thinking or understanding.

Delusional beliefs are always felt to be an absolute reality, with a conviction beyond question. There are no grey areas in thinking, everything seen only in black and white extremes. There is a lack of nuance and subtlety, with every action or remark seen in the most concrete terms. Emotional responses are either flat or extreme, with tearfulness, violence, threats or suspicions, because of damage to the subtlety and intuitive processes of the normal healthy psychological processes.

There is a lack of any clear cut boundary between a sense of personal identity and others, leading to confusion of identity, vulnerability, uncertainty where self and other begins and ends.

OBSESSIONAL ILLNESS

In obsessional illness there is loss of flexibility of attitudes and thinking. Limited thought patterns restrict understanding, undermining the development of new explorative ways of thinking. Like tunnel vision, everything in life is seen through the obsessional spyglass. The illness controls all aspects of spontaneous behaviour - work, everyday chores, eating, sleeping, sexuality, freedom of movement, relaxation and what is said, seen, or related to. This severely restricts the ability to make creative changes and shifts from one position to another. At times the body may become as rigid as the thinking, as dress and appearance reflect tight inner controls and attitudes. At times anxiety is extreme and self-confidence is low. The dominating theme is of imminent calamity unless a particular ritual is carried out to prevent or neutralise its power.

A preoccupation with cleanliness is another feature of this illness. Germs and disease are warded off in the same way as new ideas and more challenging open thinking. The mind fears what might happen if these routines are neglected, causing high levels of conflict and anxiety, to the detriment of physical and psychological health. Relaxation may be impossible.

At times, it may be impossible to stop the thoughts and rituals, fearing that this will cause irrevocable damage to a loved one, perhaps provoke illness or even death. Because the mind knows no barriers, it is also possible to believe that the obsessional ritual, in a magical way, heals or protects someone who has died or suffered in the past, sometimes a much loved pet.

Repeating the ritual is felt to ensure that any negligence (of caring) is avoided or neutralised. In some ways, the obsession resembles a penance, for not having been sufficiently loving or attentive in the past (as well as in the present). In this sense, every obsessional action has a protective function, and keeps the past alive, rather than an emerging now and a creative future. Failure to repeat the ritual, is strongly felt to be an act of omission or betrayal, leading to guilt feelings.

The obsessional driver is also full of fears. He tends to be excessively anxious, over-prudent, careful to the extreme and a menace to others. He may be full of remorse in case a shadow behind the car, means that he has run over a pigeon or hit a child, and he is never fully sure of damage he may have inadvertently committed in any area of life. Every movement of the day is dominated by the fear of his destructive omnipotence, feelings of vulnerability, and fear of danger.

Character traits which aggravate the condition
Rigid, slow, fixed attitudes are characteristic, with dislike of change. Anything new is felt to be a nuisance and a threat, unnecessarily changing the status quo and a situation of balance which has been achieved over the years. Routines and rituals may have become a way of life, dominating thought and behaviour from the moment of first waking. Decisions are only taken slowly and reluctantly, and like the future, are felt to contain unknown pitfalls and traps for the unwary rather than opportunities for growth and change.

Practical steps to improve things
Start each day in a more easy relaxed way, not falling into the same rigid routine as the day before. Try to vary your approach to each day, and if you find yourself falling into a ritual, ask yourself 'why'? Look back at the onset of any obsessional patterns and aim to understand how they first started, the emotions felt at that time, and what you may have gained by imposing them upon yourself. It is possible that you felt particularly vulnerable at the time, and developing the obsessional patterns provided you with a more stable background. You will need to look back closely at the origins as well as the present situations, in order to clarify what you are limiting now. Vary your interests, social contacts and life-style, to encourage you to make changes and to become more flexible and open in your attitudes. If you are physically fit, try taking up a new sport or exercise. You could also combine this with an artistic pursuit, to give you a different outlet of self-expression. But always stay closely in contact with others and don't choose something which will again isolate you, as this will reinforce the obsessional patterns.

Remedies to consider:-

Arsenicum

Thin and always chilly, he is typically neat and rigid in attitudes and appearance. Depressed and usually exhausted, insomnia is common, waking after midnight with obsessional worries and fears.

Calcarea

Overweight and flabby, he is always cold, and sweats profusely on the head. There are many fussy, obsessional preoccupations.

Natrum mur

Chronic insecurity is marked by lack of confidence, anxiety, and depression. There are rigid fixed thought patterns and attitudes. Exhaustion is a constant problem.

Nux vomica

A remedy for over-zealous, intense attitudes, obsessional in thinking, quick to anger, or spiteful. Self-control is weak.

Sepia

There are negative obsessional attitudes, about everything and everybody, indifferent to the family and anxious about health in general. He is exhausted, hypochondriacal and irritable, dragged down by abdominal or pelvic discomfort, problems of constipation or low backache.

PANIC ATTACKS

Severe panic can constitute a severe psychological illness which is incapacitating because the emotions and fears are powerful, overwhelming and extreme.

Levels of anxiety may be high throughout the day, often beginning on first waking, and causing total exhaustion, fear of being left alone, at times, unable to accomplish the simplest day-to-day tasks. There is apprehension of any new situations, meeting people, suddenly collapsing, feeling faint, or of illness, being in an enclosed area, for example, a lift, tunnel or subway. Others experience panic because of anxiety about their health. Panic occurs, if they feel weak or experience mild discomfort, especially a lump or a pain, often fearing a heart attack or cancer, and convinced that death is imminent. Following a physical illness some never fully recover from the fears or loss of confidence. They remain semi-invalid, convinced their days are numbered, and for this reason, they fail to fully recover. Every twinge or ache may be used as 'proof' that they are not well enough to work or travel, but fundamentally, they cannot lead a normal life because of lack of confidence. The root cause of most panic illness takes origin in a disturbance of emotional growth in childhood. There has often been damage to assertiveness, determination and drive. Feelings of anger and disagreement may have been suppressed, only to re-emerge as threats of self-destruction, complaints of being weak or ill. Frustrated drives and needs may only be expressed indirectly, building up undirected force and energy which eventually causes attacks of panic and fear.

Panic tends to alienate and can feed and intensify feelings of envy or jealousy, which may worsen any underlying psychological problems. Artistic or gifted aspects of the personality rarely flourish in these circumstances because of the limitation put on new explorative thinking and rarely realise their full potential.

Panic attacks create tension and frustration because of strong drives to be healthy and 'normal', to expand and develop, to become more independent. These needs conflict with strong infantile dependency wishes which trap the patient into a dependant, often weak, child-like role. The rigid behaviour patterns are difficult to break and may block psychological development despite strong desires to change the status quo and end a psychological impasse which causes unhappiness and frustration.

Fear of driving in traffic and on motorways are very common panic situations. Unconsciously the panic also represents powerful impulses for change, to break-away from routine and stereotyped roles, become independent and free, at the same time conflicting with dependency needs.

There may be fear of breaking a long-standing pattern, for example separating from an invalid relative who has been allowed to dominate them or fearing the commitment of a new job, relationship or marriage. Overall, there is lack of confidence about any form of change, taking on more responsibility, giving up a familiar pattern for a mature inter-dependant one. Panic attacks, may last for years and undermine the variety and richness of life.

Character traits which aggravate the condition

There is a tendency to be dependant in relationships, often the listener, but rarely the talker or spontaneous giver. This links to underlying fears of disapproval or failure, ultimately loss of love and approval, feeling not wanted, superfluous, or just a nuisance. These destructive negative attitudes may dominate every aspect of life, undermining initiative at work or in the home, limiting what is done to narrow familiar repetitive actions, but especially fearful of new challenges. He may only rarely express anger directly, tending to bury feelings, sometimes sulking, and indirectly obstructive over a minor episode for days or weeks. Open discussion of feelings, needs and ideas tends to be perfunctory and rather limited.

Practical steps to improve things

Aim to be more open and trusting, allowing yourself to talk about feelings, ideas, and directions and finding out how you react in new social situations. This will allow you to move into more challenging areas. Panic has its roots in over-dependant attitudes, usually of an infantile kind and you will need to spend time looking for these aspects of your behaviour, and finding ways to alter and mature them. It is helpful if you can discuss how you are working with your partner, a close friend, or the family. But you will need to look closely at a wide variety of situations where you experience panic or feel anxious, and slowly work at these over a period of months. Look at any areas you particularly don't want to consider or where you are inflexible, and try to reverse these. This will have a strengthening effect and help to provide insight into any areas of rigidity. Be as open as possible in all situations.

Remedies to consider:-

Aconitum

Indicated for sudden, acute attacks of panic. Moods change rapidly, restless, with everything done in a hurry. Irritability is marked, the face bright red and hot. Typical fears concern impending illness, failure at business, or death. He is fearful of shadows and the dark, going out of the house alone, crowds or queues of people. There is intolerance of draughts and cold air. Most symptoms are worse on waking and in the evening, about 10.00 pm.

Argentum nit

The remedy for an irritable, nervous temperament, full of hypochondriacal fears and compulsive thoughts. The mind is preoccupied with irrational, often bizarre depressing fears, of illness or death. The mood is one of restless anxiety, unable to relax, everything hurried. Agoraphobia (fear of open spaces), and any new or public situations are a source of fear. All symptoms are worse from heat. He is often silent and apprehensive, with a bloated sense of fullness of the stomach region. The body image is distorted.

110

Gelsemium

He is full of fears, particularly appearing in public. Tiredness and fatigue are characteristic, the eyes drooping with fatigue, the limbs weak and not reacting well. Tremor of the hands or legs is an expression of underlying tension. There is an enormous fear of failure, disapproval, making a mistake, or looking foolish. Concentration is weak due to anxiety and he finds it difficult to rest or relax.

Lycopodium

This is a useful remedy for severe anticipatory fear felt in the pit of the stomach and worse from 4.00 to 8.00 pm. He cannot relax, is irritable, impatient, often indifferent. Sudden mood changes occur and he tends always to be timid, clumsy, accident-prone, everything done in a hurry. This contributes to 'butterfly' thinking, and difficulty in concentrating, a tendency to mix up words, making frequent spelling mistakes and problems expressing himself clearly. Lack of confidence is a basic cause of many of his problems. Sweet foods are craved, especially chocolate.

111

Natrum mur   He is thin and cold, with a greasy skin, weak, depressed and quick to burst into tears. Full of fears and lacking in confidence, moods change constantly. He is always worse for consolation and reassurance, heat, or sea air. Salt is craved. There is a tendency to retain fluids, the ankles or hands swollen. Weak and exhausted, he is never at ease and relaxed in any new or social situation.

Phosphorus   A remedy for tall, impulsive, red-haired artistic people. The chest is often weak, with a tendency to wheezy breathing, shortness of breath, or asthma, especially when under pressure or stress. He is exhausted and apathetic, always chilly, yet thirsty for ice-cold drinks. There is a minimum of energy or drive, the mood irritable, fearful, restless and often unpredictable. There is a constant need for attention and reassurance, at times sitting for hours and not taking his eyes off you. An unstable circulation causes the tendency to flush up easily. He craves salt, all symptoms worse in the evening from twilight to midnight, and always better after sleep.

PARANOIA

At times, paranoid or persecutory thinking occurs in us all, especially when fatigued, under pressure, or when a series of inconvenient circumstances, such as a traffic queue, red lights, or delayed trains is in opposition to our immediate needs and wishes. Such 'normal' paranoid thinking is usually brief and superficial, often the subject of humour, and not taken too seriously. In many ways it is used mischievously, to fill in time while waiting, to cope with (and express indignation) at the frustrations and loss of time, with no loss of insight into what is reality. It does not dominate thinking or take over the priorities of the day, or interfere with the logical thought-processes of the personality.

In paranoia or a paranoid (persecutory) illness, loss of insight and an absence of playful thinking occurs. There is a profound suspicion or conviction that the recurrent frustrations of the day are part of a deliberate plot to provoke, humiliate or cause damage.

The paranoid person may experience a strong sense of being a target for orchestrated malice. At every stage of life, the smiles and body language of others are not what they seem, and felt to be a coded threat. An announcement that the train will be delayed half-an-hour is suspected of being a personal threat to provoke, warn, contact or control you directly. There is often a grandiose, element to the paranoid state of mind, leading to isolation and shunning of others. This is often based on a conviction of being chosen for an important purpose or mission, which is of such importance that it cannot be divulged to others.

There is a feeling that others, including the family and care attendant, cannot be trusted, will fail to understand or think you insane. They may betray you, fail to understand the scheme of things, the important chosen role you have been given in your mission. Royalty, government, officials, heads of state, the KGB, FBI, MI5, may all become part of the grandiose fantasy. If the delusional thinking becomes entrenched and rigid with no softening of ideas and attitudes, it may lead to a planned assault, possibly a violent murder.

A prominent figure in government or the arts may be targeted as behind the delusional beliefs and become the focus of revenge fantasies, evoking anger and resentment. These are related to feelings of infantile loss or early rejection, often linked to envy and inadequacy, which nearly always lie beneath the paranoia, with attempts to compensate for an underlying hurt, depression, or wounded narcissistic pride.

If a physical attack does occur, this may be part of a well established delusional belief and a conviction of having special powers, sometimes a message directly from God, telling of the unique (but highly rigid and intolerant) role you play in a religious cult, world politics, animal rights, the peace process or solving social problems.

The paranoid individual often feels he is the object of observation, from noise, gestures, movements, words used, each having a special significance, or he is being watched or followed, and the object of a concerted plan to destroy or damage his health and mind.

Guilt about masturbation and sexual interests, may re-appear as a paranoid belief that others know about sexual thoughts, can read his mind or his eyes, are making him the object of a homosexual smear campaign. This may be confirmed by 'voices' which call out provocative sexual remarks, either when alone, or sometimes deliberately in the presence of others, in order to embarrass him.

This sexual element may lead to delusional thinking of a homosexual nature, or it may involve prostitutes, fantasies that they are behind the messages which attack his mind, and that the only way to be free is to conduct a personal vendetta, which may lead to a series of ritualistic and violent murders.

Character traits which aggravate the condition
There is a tendency to be rigid and obsessional, usually a very private person, and a 'loner' not particularly social and outgoing, and mistrustful of others. There may have been an unhappy, difficult, loveless childhood, with failure to integrate into the family. There has usually been a profound blow to personal pride and trust when young, or loss of one or both parents at an early age. Rigid controls limit closeness, even within an established relationship, the partner always feeling at a distance, on the outside, never really getting to know him in depth.

Practical steps to improve things
The major problem in a paranoid illness is to try to develop more insight (or understanding) into the illness, because this is always lost. If you suspect you are suffering from a paranoid illness and have been diagnosed as such, or are under treatment, it is

115

important to re-establish some degree of trust in others. Trust may have been present in the past, or perhaps never occurred, because of damage to confidence as a child. But some degree is essential to allow more talking and sharing of inner feelings, to help you become more involved and secure. Try to find at least one person you can trust and believe in, really care for and relate to, in an open spontaneous way. In this way, some sharing and spontaneity can develop and you may eventually feel able to give a little of yourself from the areas where you feel hurt and vulnerable. Sharing and trust is healing, although at first it may be difficult to establish.

If you are under treatment, or in a special psychiatric unit, try to be as open as possible with your doctor, and in a group or therapy situation. Aim to develop new skills and interests which you can enjoy, where you can be more spontaneous, and can talk openly. Take regular physical exercise and eat a good quality balanced diet, to keep your body fit. Always vary your interests and physical activities, to avoid these becoming rigid or routine. Try to find a creative artistic outlet for your repressed energies and feelings, such as painting, sculpture, music or writing. Share these with others and discuss them freely. Aim to avoid keeping anything secret, trying always for an open sharing of all aspects of your mind, including your natural talents and abilities, as well as problem areas of suspicion and mistrust. If you feel you have been chosen for a special task or mission, then talk about it, and try to understand what this may symbolise and what lies behind it. Use your energy and drive for relaxation and pleasure. In this way you can limit the hold of paranoid beliefs and prevent them taking over the whole of your personality.

Remedies to consider:-

Aconitum

A remedy for sudden, acute, paranoid states of mind, with restless agitation and irritability. The face is always hot and bright red.

Aurum met

Paranoid ideas are associated with despair, severe depression, and impulses to suicide. Irritable and angry, he feels others are critical, picking on him, being offensive. Palpitations are a feature, also rheumatic joint pains. There is a sense of indignation and rage. He usually prefers to be alone.

Anacardium

There are paranoid fantasies, with a sense of unreality, anxiety and depression, quickly becoming irritable. He feels he has a double, or is surrounded by enemies, persecuted and followed. Pessimistic, he foresees only danger and misfortune in the future. The memory is poor. There is a sensation of a tight band, around the body, or he feels as if he has a foreign body, or splinter inside him. Odd hallucinatory smells, especially of charred or burned wood.

117

Baryta carb

A remedy for states of confusion and depression. Timid, fearful of all new social contacts, it is particularly useful for senile delusional states. The memory is weak.

Belladonna

Indicated for confused, agitated, paranoid states. The face is hot, congested, dark-red or purple, eyes dilated, neck vessels beating violently, the pulse racing. He is violent, due to paranoid hallucinations, often fearful of being attacked by dogs, other animals, ghosts or phantoms. He is always terrified of being alone.

Cannabis ind

Indicated for confused, excitable, paranoid states of mind. He imagines he is being attacked or robbed, the house burgled, or that he is about to die. At other times he is tense and angry, about to explode like a bomb or damage buildings. There is profound anguish and despair. A spaced-out sensation, makes time pass very slowly, at times seeming extended or endless.

Hyoscyamus   A remedy for overactive states of mind, with restless agitation dominated by fear. The pupils are dilated. Constantly talking and hallucinated, he is mistrustful of his medicines (believes they are poisoned). Paranoid ideas provoke anxieties of being attacked. He is suspicious and mistrustful of everyone.

Kali Brom   There are acute delusional fears of being pursued by the police, his life is in danger, friends are against him or have deserted him, he has been chosen to be the victim of divine vengeance. Agitated and fearful, he attempts to throw himself from a window. Moods are variable. At times he feels timid, depressed, fearful, and he may become violent.

Lachesis   For talkative, arrogant, weeping, excitable states of mind, often frightened, irritable, suspicious or jealous. He is convinced that death is imminent, with many paranoid ideas. Intolerant of tight clothes, all symptoms are worse after sleep.

119

Plumbum met   For weak, exhausted states, pale, drawn, and emaciated. Paranoid delusions, with fear of being attacked or poisoned. There are violent outbursts of rage and hallucinations. The mood is often one of depression, apathy or indifference. Colicky abdominal pains are characteristic with weakness or paralysis of certain muscles e.g. wrist drop. He tends to lose weight, and there may be persistent constipation. The hands tend to develop a tremor.

Rhus tox   For restless, fearful, paranoid or irritable states of mind, fearing that others want to harm him, are plotting, or following him. There is a mood of despair and pessimism. All symptoms are worse at night, when resting. He feels better for warmth, heat and movement.

PHOBIAS

These relate to everyday situations where there is an overwhelming amount of fear and apprehension. Typical examples are:- fear of being trapped, locked in a cupboard or lift, travel, especially a long bridge, tunnel, the underground, or a plane or the train. Also when it is impossible to get off immediately and long distance journeys with increasing distance from home. Phobias usually relate to childhood insecurity, often because the parents themselves were nervous in similar situations, and their anxiety and uncertainty was communicated to the child.

In all phobias, there is trapped emotional energy, which cannot be allowed to emerge spontaneously, finding an exit as symptoms of anticipatory anxiety or fear. Phobic symptoms tend to limit both movement and levels of individual personal achievement.

A phobia is nearly always a symptom of an inner conflict. Fear of being shut-in, trapped, or sometimes locked-out, reflects the levels of tension felt by the personality, as drive, ambition, and libido, or any motivating force for change and independence are kept under lock and key.

In many ways, the phobic symptoms come to symbolise areas of the person which are blocked and denied, the feared cupboards and tunnels, reflecting attitudes of mind, and used as part of its defence mechanism. These are particularly active against feelings of vulnerability, dependency, sensitivity and need. As the blocked individual drive symbolically bangs on the door in anger and protest at its imprisonment, it is often this

121

which gives the experience of panic, fear, and anxiety.

For many phobics, anger rather than fear, is nearest the surface, for example, when held up in a queue at the supermarket check-out. The waiting comes to represent psychologically being fenced in or blocked, within the rigid inner boundaries of the phobic problem. The frustrations, anxiety, and impatience felt, causes intense anxiety, a sense of short-fuse impatience and at times, almost violent anger. These blocked aspects of individuality lead to powerful emotions, feeling frightened and enraged at being thwarted, close to violent anger and loss of control.

Parts of the self want to break out from the phobia and develop, find their place in the world, become free and a person, with more creative self-expression, satisfaction and happiness. These drives for growth and change, are also intolerant and impatient, resenting the brakes applied to them. Such feelings are usually kept denied, suppressed and largely unconscious. When they threaten to emerge the emotions feel raw and strong because they have been denied any form of outlet over the years. The underlying drives for change have often grown in strength, despite the limitations set on them by the phobic process, and it is their increased demands for greater self-expression, growth and change which causes panic and phobia.

Fear of open spaces (agoraphobia) is frequently a fear of being swallowed-up by the vastness of the square or landscape. Sometimes a ribbon-like road seems to go on endlessly and emphasises underlying feelings of being small and insignificant, at the same time, usually referring to feelings of need.

Sometimes the phobias become obsessional to the point of becoming psychotic or delusional in type. One example is fear of travelling by train to the office, in case minute pieces of broken glass, or other small objects such as dust or dirt, are blown in through the open carriage window, damaging the eyes, and causing blindness. This degree of severe obsessional phobia can be best understood by seeing the eye as a symbol of the personal self (ego) or 'I', and the glass as disapproval for thinking and looking (or wanting to). In others, voyeuristic sexual fantasies and looking have been replaced by fear of blindness for daring to think sexual thoughts, usually linked to masturbation. These fantasies may have developed into a phobia because at the time they originated there was a major trauma within the family, perhaps a divorce or separation, sometimes a serious illness or death. This combination can sometimes lead to guilt feelings and psychological blockage, the feelings becoming displaced and unacceptable, but expressed in a symbolic way as a phobia or blockage. Feelings of guilt, frustration and inadequacy, limit personal freedom, the ability to make changes, and creative self-expression.

Character traits which aggravate the condition

There is a tendency to control all emotions and to avoid spontaneity, feeling vulnerable and insecure. A major factor is keeping feelings secret, not being open enough or sharing. This may centre around any feelings and emotions, but particularly needs, love and affection, anger or resentment, also sexual interests and drive.

Practical steps to improve things

Aim to be more open with others. In at least one area, try to be giving and spontaneous, not holding back or blocking what you really think and feel, where in the past you have been on the defensive. Map out your main phobic areas, and how they started. It is helpful to look back at the key events which were happening in your life, and try to make some very honest links with your feelings at that time, and the development of the phobic symptoms. There is often a link which you may have forgotten or repressed, but it should be possible to find it if you allow yourself to free-associate and to relax. It may take several weeks to make the link, but be relaxed about it, and don't try too hard to make changes, as this will only raise anxiety levels or block the associations you need to make. The key link sometimes occurs as a result of a dream, so try to understand them, as you work on yourself. Once you have found more recent links with the onset of a particular phobic area, try to think back to childhood to see if you were fearful at that time. Re-examine the key events which occurred at the time when you started to become more inward looking, secretive or fearful, less spontaneous and out-going. At the same time, clarify your present aims and directions and how you are blocking them.

Remedies to consider:-

Argentum nit
Hypochondriacal, depressive thoughts provoke phobic anxiety problems. Weak and irritable, often dragged down by moods of fear and anxiety, there is a preoccupation with fears of illness. Obsessional thoughts dominate each corner of the road or building, thinking about a certain angle, that the building may fall. All symptoms are worse from heat.

Belladonna
Thoughts are rapid, often of a hypochondriacal nature, with confusion and disorientation. He is easily irritated, moods shifting from laughter and being over-talkative, to domination by fear.

Borax
For anxiety with agitation, sensitive to all forms of sudden noise. All symptoms are worse from a downward motion, with fear of falling, anxiety going down an escalator or stairs, in a plane. He dislikes swings, a rocking chair, or anything which causes a forward motion. Indifferent to others. Most symptoms are worse in the late evening.

Calcarea

Indicated when the person is fair, overweight, apathetic, chilly, weak and cold, a tendency to sweat on the head. Anxiety with palpitations is common and he is often restless and irritable. All symptoms are worse after any form of mental effort. The overall mood is one of depression and sadness. Obsessed by detail, he can sit for hours counting pins or preoccupied with trivial object.

Calcarea phos

For a dark complexioned, thin person. Indifference is marked with irritability. Depressed, fearful, weak, he always feels worse from damp cool air.

Carboneum sulph

A remedy for depressed, irritable moods. Concentration is poor. Vague, the memory is weak.

Cicuta virosa

Anxiety with sweating is marked, with agitation and overactivity. He trembles with tension, and the mood is one of sadness. There are fears of death. He is suspicious, lacking confidence, and prefers to be alone.

126

Digitalis   There are feelings of guilt and fear of death. He lacks confidence, anticipating failure or criticism. Moods are tearful, irritable and depressed. Palpitations and a sense of oppression in the heart are other indications for this remedy.

Graphites   There are many obsessional fears, the chest tight. He is restless, depressed and weeping, often fearing death. The moods vary, at times, excitable, hesitant, or timid. Music often causes a mood of tearful despondency.

Ignatia   For phobias associated with grief or loss. Intolerant of any form of contradiction, the least criticism causes anger or irritability. He tends to blame himself, tearful, impatient, lacking confidence. Depressed and sighing, he prefers his own company, often weak and exhausted. The stomach feels as if it has a hole in it.

Kali arsen

A remedy for restless, agitated, phobic states with confusion of mind. The skin is irritated with a dry eczema, grey and dirty-looking and often infected.

Lycopodium

Most of the fears are about the future. His mind is always tilted forward, thinking about what might happen next, unconcerned with the present. He is accident-prone and takes risks to gain approval and to be noticed. This tends to isolate him from others and adds to lack of confidence.

Natrum carb

For depressed tearful moods of despondency and hopelessness. Anxiety with restlessness is common. He is irritable, frightened by the least noise. Worse for music or noise, he is also irritated by bright lights.

Phosphorus

The individual is tall and thin, with a weak chest. He is popular and likes people, but can drive them away by his endless need for attention and reassurance. He is easily frightened, apathetic, with no inclination to work or study. Time passes too slowly.

Platinum

A remedy where arrogant pride is a predominant character trait, looking down on others with contempt. They seem small, inferior or insignificant. At the same time, he is fearful, insecure, full of anxieties concerning death or that some disaster is imminent. Restless, irritable, depressed, and weeping, moods change quickly from laughter to tears. Objects are also distorted, either too narrow or small. He is terrified, because of a conviction, that something is about to happen which will cause him harm. The mood is always negative and pessimistic.

Psorinum

A remedy for depressed, tearful states of fear, preoccupied with death, fire, or business failure. Stubborn and obstinate, there are sudden mood changes. He is disinclined to work and dislikes washing. He worries about his poor memory, social impressions and the impact made on others, always chilly, even in summer.

129

Sepia

Usually indicated for a tall person with dark hair and eyes, with a tendency to sweat. He is irritable, quick to anger, tearful, gloomy and pessimistic. There is a chilly emotional indifference to those loved best, distant and apathetic. The predominant mood is of depression. He can't think or collect his thoughts and has few ambitions. Exhausted and fearful, only dancing or rapid exercise improves the condition. He often finds thunder exhilarating.

Stramonium

Fear dominates all aspect of the personality, with a most intense and phobic state of anxiety with confusion. There is fear of dogs and all liquids, especially water, and even the thought of it is disturbing. He may be restless or excitable, often noisy. Delusional convictions lead to a phobic preoccupation with insects or small animals, which he sees all around the room or on the bed. He is despairing and fearful, terrified if left alone. In many ways he is emotionally like a small, angry, terrified child. All symptoms are worse after sleep.

PSYCHOSIS

Essentially, psychosis is a severe illness of the mind, where there is alienation from others, due to a break with reality. This severs the links of understanding between self and others, causing misperception, distorted thinking, communication problems, impaired judgement and understanding. The ability to clarify and differentiate between the outer world of reality and the inner complex of imagination and fantasy is vital for psychological health. In a psychotic illness, this is lost, at times totally, although it is often rationalised by a delusional process, which adds to confusion.

The psychotic or divided mind withdraws into its own world of omnipotent fantasy. It fails to perceive others as separate, but only as an extension of an inner imaginative world. Because the thought processes and emotions of the psychotic mind are completely omnipotent and powerful, it also leads to beliefs that others are threatening and potentially dangerous. A profound sense of fear and mistrust develops, often feelings of intense jealousy and suspicion, in many instances associated with sexual anxieties. There is interference with normal thinking, causing a distorted interpretation of others and their motivations, and an impaired understanding of their intentions and actions.

The exact cause of a psychotic illness is not always known, but it often follows a period of prolonged pressure and stress. Among the most common causes are:- overwork at college or university, a poor diet with inadequate rest or sleep, isolation or alienation from others. The pressure of college work may be highlighted by an insensitive, demanding family which takes

131

success for granted, or a sibling may have a natural high academic ability adding to pressures to succeed. Feelings of being unable to attain family expectations may lead to depression and dread of failure. It is common to feel that the family has been let down, or failure will never be accepted and forgiven. If the family has made financial sacrifices to support the student through his studies, this adds to guilt feelings, with a hopeless sense of failure and futility. Other causes of a psychotic illness include :- the breakdown of a relationship, failure to establish a close relationship with the opposite sex because of social inexperience or shyness, and homosexuality. Feelings are aggravated, pressures intensified, if there is an older or younger sibling, who has a successful and stable relationship, intensifying competitive feelings, guilt, resentment, envy and jealousy.

As a result of tension and fear, there is a build-up of feelings, which cannot be immediately resolved because of immaturity and the limitations of the people concerned. A potential emotional time-bomb occurs. This may continue to build-up inside until it cannot be contained, causing withdrawal and alienation. An accumulation of self-destructive thoughts and impulses, tends to dominate thinking, and these may eventually lead to inappropriate psychotic behaviour and beliefs, at times to an overdose or a successful suicide.

Avoidance of others, solitary, self-contained pursuits, being a 'loner', may have been a long-standing defence against feelings of nervousness, tension and inadequacy. Such tendencies may have been intensified by a lack of social skills and experience. Shyness, and reluctance to admit or talk about personal feelings, may have been an added factor, leading to remoteness, a preference for solitude, a world of speculation and theory, religion and philosophy, rather than open and meaningful sharing experiences with others.

The psychotic withdrawal into fantasy makes him feel constantly threatened or under attack. Everyone seems to be an enemy and no one can be fully trusted. For this reason he feels vulnerable and at times lonely, with few or no true friends. In order to survive he must be on guard all the time, convinced he is unloved, others are plotting against him and talking about him in a denigratory way. He feels others know his most private thoughts and feelings including sexual inclinations, and can omnipotently read his mind. Others are felt to control his thoughts, or send thoughts and ideas into his mind, often of a threatening or obscene nature.

It is not difficult to see that at the root of many forms of psychotic illness, there are profound problems of closeness and trust, and also difficulties in coming to terms with closeness, and sexual feelings.

The delusional process gives the psychotic a framework to understand the external world, a way of rationalising what is happening. It gives a sense to the fragmented thoughts, inconsistent impulses and drives he experiences. He may believe he has been chosen to play a unique world role to put the universe in order, with secret links to God, his chosen son, or related to a world leader of power and influence. At the same time, he is often preoccupied with both sex and religion, feeling guilty for his 'sins'. All of this reflects underlying anxiety about acceptance, success, status, often guilt about masturbation and sexual impulses.

133

Certainty is a marked feature of every psychotic illness, with rigid extremes of thinking, and total conviction beyond doubt of the validity of the delusional beliefs. Because words and phrases are broken down and used in a concrete unimaginative way, this may destroy their expressive, poetic or symbolic sense, undermining fluency and creative self-expression.

Character traits which aggravate the condition
A tendency to be quiet, withdrawn and shy. Little opportunity is allowed for spontaneous free-expression of feelings and emotion. Anger is rarely shown, tending to emerge as sulky frustration, and rage directed inwards as silent provocation. It may also occur as a physical symptom such as asthma, stomach cramps or vomiting, rather than being openly expressed.

There is a preoccupation with the world of fantasy, fascinated by odd weird ideas which cannot ever come to fruition because they are not based on a reality premise. Personal relationships are often limited, especially with the opposite sex. Masturbation is usually misunderstood and a major area of guilt. Homosexual fantasies are the other important area of sexual guilt and preoccupation, which is equally destructive.

Practical steps to improve things

If you have been diagnosed as having a psychotic illness, or are under treatment, it is possible to combine homoeopathic treatment with the orthodox approach, also with counselling or psychotherapy. If you are experiencing voices or have any unusual convictions or beliefs, you need to understand why they have developed and to discuss them openly. At the same time, try to establish some genuine areas of trust, friendship and sharing. Because of damage to basic insight and understanding as a result of the illness, it is likely that your knowledge of what has triggered off the illness is rather fragmentary. But once you have found someone you can trust, perhaps a friend or counsellor, try to look back at the last time you were completely well, and clarify in detail the events which led to your breakdown. These may involve an area of emotional tension and pressure, perhaps an acute rejection or disappointment, but try to get this clear in your mind. As you work at your feelings, try also to look back at any similar incidents in your childhood when you were thrown off course by a trauma, time of uncertainty, or heightened emotional tensions. Clarify these particular happenings in your life, and how they affected you, your reactions, and subsequent development.

Psychotic illness is curable and it is possible to make a full and lasting recovery from this kind of mental illness.

Remedies to consider:-

Aconitum

For acute, restless, excitable states of mind. Moods are variable, but anxiety levels are always at a high level. At times he becomes depressed or aggressive, demanding and impatient. He is fearful and timid, frightened of the dark or shadows. An acute manic state may develop. The condition is aggravated by music, and also worse for exposure to draughts of cold, dry air.

Anacardium

A remedy for hallucinated states, with inappropriate responses to questions, the mood variable. At times he may be anxious and depressed, fearful of the future, memory and concentration poor. The body image is also affected, with a delusion concerning a hoop or tight band encircling him, having a foreign body inside the abdomen, or convinced he has a double.

Baptisia

He complains of weakness, poor concentration, feels sleepy and apathetic. The mind is agitated and confused, all the emotions variable. At times he may become convinced he has a double, or has

136

separated into pieces, and heseeks ways to re-unite the pieces of his being. The breath is typically foul and fetid.

Belladonna

A remedy for violent, excitable, hallucinated, hyper-active psychotic states. There is a desire to bite, tearing at the sheets or clothes. The face is flushed dark red or purple, pupils dilated, the neck vessels visibly pulsating. He is confused and agitated, hyper-sensitive to bright lights, cold air, touch, loud noise, tending to develop spasmodic pains in any part of the body, particularly the throat, gall-bladder, stomach or kidney.

Cannabis ind

Indicated for excitable, laughing, talkative, psychotic conditions, fixed ideas and hallucinations. He is convinced he has a double. Moods are changeable, from laughter to tears. He hears music, bells playing, the mind clouded and vague. Dizziness with vertigo is a feature and time passes very slowly.

Hyoscyamus

For highly excitable, violent and often destructive psychotic states. He is restless, suspicious, and tends to talk rapidly. Moods are variable. As a result of continued tension, muscular contractions, fits or spasms may occur. There are many delusional fears of being poisoned, with an aversion to water, and all forms of liquid.

Petroleum

For irritable states of mind, quick to anger. The skin is dry, encrusted, itchy and sensitive, tending to crack or becomes infected, discharging a clear liquid. He is always hungry, the stomach feels empty and he is often cold in localised areas of the body. Hallucinations develop, and he is convinced he has a double. Because of the mental confusion, he becomes confused or lost, often in quite familiar surroundings.

Stramonium

For fearful, agitated states of confusion. He fears he is being attacked by dogs, and has a marked aversion to water or any form of fluid. At times the delusional process causes his though processes to become incoherent and muddled. He may see visual hallucinations of animals, phantoms, insects in his room. Tearful and depressed, he gazes out at his surroundings with fear.

PUERPERAL PSYCHOSIS

This is a severe form of mental illness, which only occurs after childbirth. It does not develop at other times, and does not necessarily recur following a subsequent pregnancy, although there is a slightly higher risk. The cause is unknown, but the illness may be associated with stress, before or during the pregnancy, excessive fatigue, and hormonal imbalance. The previous personality has usually been quite healthy, strong, happy and outgoing, with no previous history of an earlier breakdown or nervous problems.

In the past, there may have been a tendency to keep anxieties under wraps, to over-protect the partner from fears or doubts, sometimes avoiding a particular problem area, because of not wanting to worry him. A facade of being happy and anxiety-free may become a source of guilt, feeling that there are no real or major problems. Doubts or difficulties are felt to be of her own making and that in many ways, life is perfect or near ideal. Feeling loved yet somehow not happy, she may feel she can't discuss it because there are no reasons to feel unhappy. She may also miss her previous job and friends but can't tell anyone because she feels guilty that there is no logical cause for her tears or low moods. As a result these emotions become buried, and once denied, can become a source of psychological illness at the end of the pregnancy.

Coming to terms with ambivalent or mixed feelings during the pregnancy is not easy for any woman, yet this is a time when illogical feelings do come up to the surface and seem to make no sense, because she has every reason to be happy. A tendency to withdraw or to isolate herself from friends and family may occur, perhaps hidden under a pretence of being too busy or 'tired'. The mother may try to hide her emotional difficulties, to all outward appearances, happy and confident, but this also saps her energy and adds to the natural fatigue she feels, causing additional anxiety. She may feel unable to cope with the daily household chores, dreading an illness and fearing the worst, but still not speak about it because she does not want to worry her partner or the family.

Initially, the mother may appear a little jaded, less enthusiastic than usual, but otherwise well. Eventually the underlying and unspoken areas of doubt begin to form clusters of anxiety, irritability, suspicion and doubt, especially when under strain, at the end of the day, and when she feels tired. If none of these feelings have been talked through during pregnancy, there may be an increase in tension a week or more after the birth. The mood may change, as she is unable to relax or sleep, becoming restless, nervous and irritable. Eventually the first sign of the psychotic illness manifests as a delusional idea, perhaps feeling watched, that she is about to be attacked, the baby is not hers, or has been changed in some way. In addition, she may feel a nuisance and a failure, her mood varying from abject tearful misery, depression and melancholia with suicidal thoughts, to excitable moods, when she runs out of the house, perhaps taking the baby and the other children to a safe haven, sometimes driving miles to her parent's home, in order to feel 'safe'.

She may suspect her husband, or mother-in-law, of being involved in a plot to wreck her health, to undermine her personality, as the destructive nature of the psychotic process becomes externalised (through projection), onto close members of the family. In a severe psychotic illness, she may pose a risk to the baby if she feels it is 'evil' and not her own, is destroying her marriage and her sanity, draining all her strength, the basic cause of her problems and the reason why she is being 'watched' or 'followed'.

The birth process and delivery may have been perfectly 'normal', followed by healthy breast-feeding, or sometimes a curious reluctance to nurse the baby and failure to establish close psychological bonding. In some cases the failure to bond has followed a period of separation immediately after birth because the baby was immature and underweight, requiring an incubator or surgery, or the mother was perhaps too ill and toxic after the delivery, which kept her separate from the baby during the critical early days when bonding occurs.

During the treatment of any puerperal psychosis, it often becomes clear that there has been a long-standing damage to confidence, which has been present at quite a deep level within the personality, but never previously declared or admitted. Where this is an underlying factor, the psychotic illness may have been triggered by high levels of emotion and stress associated with pregnancy and the delivery, especially if it was at all prolonged or difficult. If the upbringing of the mother was narrow and over-strict, this may also contribute to narrow rigid attitudes in later life, creating conflict and doubts which are not easily expressed or talked about.

Case report

One mother, who had experienced a rigid, over-strict religious upbringing, developed a puerperal psychosis after her third child. She felt guilty about occasional anal intercourse with her husband, but could not discuss it with him. She did not enjoy this particular form of intimacy, but knew that her husband did, and felt in a turmoil for months, unable to talk to anyone about it. In every other aspect, their relationship was close, supportive, harmonious and balanced. If her husband had been aware of her feelings about this particular form of sexuality, he would not have continued.

Problems often arise, when parts of the self become deflected, pushed down, and then denied. This is always undesirable, but particularly at times of fatigue and pressure, as occurs after a birth, and most of all after a first baby. When underlying feelings are intense, without access to dialogue and sharing, they may revolt against the conscience or conscious controls, and find an exit in the form of a puerperal psychotic illness.

After the illness, many mothers are more mature, more relaxed than in the past, and seem to have moved forward in basic confidence and personal development. During the acute psychotic stage of the illness, hospitalisation may be necessary to protect the mother and child from the intensity and drive of the delusional process.

In addition to the homoeopathic medicines, sedation and orthodox drugs may be required. These can be prescribed together, in total safety, without any risk of side-effects or interaction occurring.

Character traits which aggravate the condition

Narrow and rigid attitudes, keep feelings and emotions inside, failing to talk about them spontaneously or in sufficient depth and making it difficult for confidence and maturity to occur. Many of the difficulties may be hidden under a facade that everything is 'alright', when the woman is really feeling anxious, uncertain and depressed.

Practical steps to improve things

Try to be open with your partner, but also with others, including friends, the family and your children. Aim to overcome infantile inhibitions by sharing and giving out feelings, at the same time listening to the needs of others. Avoid a passive position of just being a listener without contributing. Throughout the pregnancy be as relaxed as you can, giving yourself regular rest breaks, sharing the chores with your partner, and not running yourself down, either physically by being Mrs. Perfect, or psychologically, by unreasonable self-criticism and feelings of guilt. If you feel tired don't be afraid to say so. Always discuss any feelings of doubt, apprehension, tension or depression with your partner as soon as they occur. If you are not able to talk and discuss with him because of limitations within the relationship, then talk to your doctor, a close female friend, your midwife or health visitor. Should doubts occur concerning basic trust, or you feel under attack and in a 'siege' situation involving you or the new baby, then discuss it immediately with your partner or close family.

Remedies to consider:-

Aurum met   A remedy for severe puerperal psychotic depressed states with determined impulse to suicide. The woman feels very despondent, with a marked sense of indescribable anguish, due to tension. She is often extremely irritable, hypersensitive to noise, touch, or bright lights. Heart palpitations are a feature, also rheumatic or arthritic pains.

Baryta carb   Indicated when the woman is sad, dejected, and tearful, convinced she is going to die. Fearful as well as irritable, she is utterly despairing about the future.

Belladonna   The woman is overactive and aggressive, inclined to bite or attack. The face is red and hot, the pupils dilated, neck and head arteries clearly seen to be beating violently. She is restless, deluded at times, talkative, intolerant of noise and light.

Camphor   For restless excitement with agitation. The woman may foam at the mouth with rage and fury, wanting to kill someone. There are wild delusional impulses, agonizing fear and depression.

Cimicifuga

A remedy for puerperal delusional states with anxiety. There is a tearful, sighing depression. Talking and agitated, the mind runs from one idea to another, as if enclosed within a thick fog, a heavy lead weight on the head. She may become incoherent. Overactivity leads to exhaustion. Moods are changeable, the fears endless. She is suspicious, with hallucinations of insects or small animals, running around the room.

Crotalus horrib

There is an excessive, very excitable mood with delusions. All symptoms are worse at night. She is depressed, apprehensive indifferent. All the emotions are very variable.

Cuprum met

Moods change from laughter to tears, with extremes of anxiety and fear. She can quickly change and become irritable or angry. There is an overall lack of interest and drive, a sense of apathy. Violent cramps or convulsions may occur, causing exhaustion of mind and body. There is extreme hypersensitivity, both physically and mentally.

145

Hyoscyamus

A remedy for highly excitable, restless, violent mental states, attacking others, at times over-talkative, out of control and manic. Inappropriate movements or gestures may occur, related to the delusional process. The remedy is particularly indicated for extreme states of anxiety and restlessness. At other times, and in complete contrast, the woman lies inert, apparently lethargic or in a state of stupor.

Kali brom

Indicated for violent mental states of confusion with constant agitation or restlessness. There may be auditory or visual hallucinations, often persecutory in type. The mother feels followed or threatened by others, with paranoid delusions, fearing they are conspiring to kill her, or she has been singled out for divine vengeance. The underlying mood is one of severe depression with total despondency.

Kali carb

There is a fearful, changeable state of mind, with varying irritable moods. The woman is antagonistic, fearful of the future, lacking in confidence, and easily

146

frightened. She may experience visual hallucinations, e.g. that there is another person in the room, or she is being tormented by imaginary images, fearful of the least noise and of being touched. At other times she can be apathetic and depressed.

Lycopodium   A remedy for milder depressed states. The mother is fearful and irritable and in a state of anguish. She may misuse words or mispronounce them. Her thoughts are muddled and confused. There is an aggravation in the late afternoon or early evening from 4.00 to 8.00 pm. She often craves chocolate or sweet foods.

Platinum   A useful remedy for visual disturbances, when everything seems distorted, small or inferior, remote and far away. She feels larger than others and behaves in an arrogant, superior, deluded way. Others are looked down on with contempt and pride, wanting to have nothing to do with them. This is a reflection of her profound loss of confidence and self-esteem. At other times she is depressed and weeping, fearing death, anxious and irritable. She may also have an overwhelming impulse to kill herself or the young baby.

Sepia

A valuable remedy for puerperal mental states where there is a combination of depression with delusional beliefs. The mother looks sallow, almost yellow in colour, the skin oily. She is profoundly tired and indifferent to the baby. There may be delusional attempts to harm the child, particularly if she believes it has been changed, is in some way 'evil', or at the root of her suffering.

Stramonium

Indicated for wild, excitable, noisy states of weeping, terror or laughter. At times she becomes despairing or incoherent, particularly fearing dogs and being bitten. Depression leads her to feel life is over. There may be both visual and tactile hallucinations, as if insects are walking over the skin. Muscular spasms or grimacing are also part of the hyper-excitable mental state. There is a profound aversion to all fluids, and the thought of water may lead to extreme restlessness. She can become aggressive if restrained.

Veratrum alb   The body is ice-cold, covered with sweat, the mother weak and complaining of burning pains. She is deluded, with grandiose ideas, at times haughty and superior. At other times, she becomes irritable and quick to anger, wanting to strike out. There is a sense of despair and failure, inconsolable, as if she has lost everything. Tearful anxiety and depression dominates most of her moods.

Veratrum viride   A remedy for irritable, depressive states of mind, with impulses to strike out, hit or kick. There may be fear of death. Nausea and vomiting are associated with the mental state.

Zincum met   Indicated when the woman is over-talkative, irritable, and depressed. She feels weak, but the lower limbs or feet are constantly agitated, fidgety and restless. There may be a tremor of the hands. Jerky spasms of muscular groups occur in the limbs, due to the hyper-excitable nervous state and leading to uncontrollable movements or loss of co-ordination.

SCHIZOPHRENIA

Schizophrenia, or 'split mind' is a form of acute psychosis in young adults. It is often recurrent, and leads to psychotic delusional beliefs, states of fear, confusion, and hallucinations. There may be periods of withdrawal, apathy or inactivity, spending long hours alone, preoccupied with fantasy, feelings of frustration or depression. At other times flights of fantasy occur, with overactivity leading to manic behaviour, which cannot always be controlled in the home. When this happens, a period of hospitalisation is often necessary. At other times, the schizophrenic may be more relaxed, in touch with reality and having insight into his condition, able to converse and relate in a healthy way, perhaps talk about his periods of crisis and why they happen. This is always a positive encouraging sign and shows that a healthy part of the mind is present and can function perfectly well, as long as it is not overwhelmed by the psychotic process at times of stress or emotional upheaval. Periods of more balanced thinking, reacting and insight, as well as delusional beliefs, is always positive and suggests the possibility of a full cure.

The onset of schizophrenia often occurs without warning of the pent-up emotions and conflicts which eventually precipitate a breakdown. The acute illness is usually preceded by a period of intense pressure at college or university, not coping with revision and exams at the end of the term. A student may have obsessionally worked non-stop for weeks before an examination, draining all reserves, leaving him jaded, fearful, and exhausted. Others have neglected all regular course work until a few weeks before an end-of-year test, leading inevitably to poor grades or failure, the possibility of losing a grant, having to abandon the course, or spend extra time at college, rather than moving on. Others may have experienced an earlier disappointment or rejection within a close relationship, either in reality, or sometimes in total fantasy. A common problem is failure to establish a close friendship or involvement with the opposite sex.

One young schizophrenic in her early 20's described how students would provoke her at college, telling her she was attractive and 'sexy', but none ever followed it up or asked her out. None of the boys at college seemed to really want to get to know her, and she was left feeling angry, disappointed and sexually frustrated.
The previous personality of the schizophrenic has often lacked confidence, shy with others, especially the opposite sex. There is a tendency to withdraw, becoming quiet, over-anxious, over-reacting or guilty about sexual jokes and discussions. It may not be easy to talk and share with others, holding back or slow to interact because of shyness, especially in group situations. He may form isolated friendships with quiet, withdrawn or intellectual types, the relationships kept very private. Friendships tend to occur with others who have had a similar psychotic experience and a breakdown, or a very narrow specialised band of interests.

Because he lacks a firm sense of reality, the schizophrenic tends to become fascinated by philosophy. He may speculate endlessly about the nature and meaning of life or religion, rather than having a firm and solid base for belief and faith. At the same time he can become concerned about reality needs and issues, finding a job, earning money, being independent, how to afford a room or a flat, find a girl-friend. Many of the preoccupations which take over his attention and thought processes are rooted in infantile needs, and relate to feelings of vulnerability, fear of destructive omnipotent fantasies. The healthy side of the personality may at the same time be concerned with quite valid social issues, reflecting a caring, healthy side of his nature. This is sometimes shown by intense concern about any form of exploitation or suffering, particularly of animals, an endangered species, perhaps the plight of whales. Concern and positive intentions may also be shown towards any group of people who are being persecuted or in need, reflecting a deep sensitive awareness of human need and suffering. The way such concern is expressed is often excessive, or vague, speculative and unrealistic, tending to highlight anxiety and fear. Because of fragmentation, and the unreal nature of the schizophrenic thought process, the ability to mobilise the mind into a coherent form of action or strategy may be impossible. This is because all activity and commitment has to be approved by the inner fantasy world, rather than the needs of reality, and inevitably this causes hesitancy, confusion, or a tendency to identify with those in need. Because of the concrete nature of his thinking, the schizophrenic is never quite sure whether he is the victim and at risk, the aggressor, or the concerned helper trying to resolve the situation. At times he may feel identified with all three aspects in a very real way, causing divided feelings of fear and utter terror, aggression or despondency.

Character traits which aggravate the condition

There is a tendency to withdraw from others, to hold feelings in. Shyness and passivity are common features. Illness occurs, combined with failure to communicate needs and feelings. This leads to an accumulation of emotions which begin to act independently from the rest of the personality. Anger and negative feelings are usually kept hidden or denied, and this causes them to fester or to find an alternative outlet, as in destructive jealousy or envy. This may then lead on to guilt, a sense of failure or feelings of inadequacy. The schizophrenic usually lacks the ability for sustained drive, because he anticipates failure, and tends to shun all social or competitive situations.

Practical steps to improve things

The ideal is to prevent the condition occurring, by the family supporting open self-expression and dialogue at an early stage of development. Any child who has a tendency to become isolated self-absorbed, obsessional in any way, a loner or 'odd' should be seen by a psychologist and assessed at an early date. It is far better to have a period of counselling or therapy before the illness develops rather than after, but this is not always possible because the family fails to perceive that the child or adolescent is at risk. If you have been diagnosed as schizophrenic, you will need help to improve your condition and to regain insight. It is often best to combine homoeopathy with a period of counselling or psychotherapy, but try to find someone you like, trust and feel you can work with. This is often best approached during a period of relative calm, rather then during a time of acute crisis or activity, either when you are under treatment in hospital, or when you have been discharged.

Remedies to consider:-

Arsenicum

There are many fears, including being alone and the dark. The mood is often one of tearful depression, anguish and despair. Restless feelings may cause a sense of becoming overwhelmed. Mental agitation is marked, with fastidious, obsessional patterns of thinking and acting. At times there may be violent, psychotic delusional states, which may lead to a suicide attempt. Symptoms are worse from 1-3.00 am. and burning pains are a typical feature. He is always chilly and better for heat.

Belladonna

For violent, restless, states of fury and agitation, the face red and hot, pupils dilated, the pulse full and rapid, with obvious pulsation of the neck carotid arteries. A confused, deluded state of terror exists, at times screaming with terror or crying out with fear. He feels threatened by the presence of others, and has hallucinations of people or animals in the room, who he then tends to fight off. There is intolerance of noise and bright lights. Vertigo with dizziness is a common complaint.

Hyoscyamus

The remedy is indicated for extreme restless states, becoming hypermanic and uncontrollable. Deluded, suspicious, jealous, and often violent, he feels poisoned by his medicines. He makes many inappropriate gestures or actions, the mood abruptly changing from terror to laughter. Over-talkative, he is also irritable and may become violent. Muscular spasms occur, with repetitive tics, mannerisms and odd jerky movements. All symptoms are worse at night, and when lying in bed. The patient feels weak and exhausted, unable to control his thought processes or find adequate words to express himself.

Lycopodium

He is confused, especially at night, with irrational, delusional beliefs, preoccupied with the meaning of life and religion. He experiences a frightening sense of unreality, as if split off from the rest of his body. Excitable, moods quickly change from inappropriate laughter to tears, irritability, or violence. The underlying mood is one of depression, at times suspicion, and often using inappropriate or meaningless words.

155

He feels very vulnerable, and dislikes being alone. Memory is weak, all symptoms worse from 4-8.00 pm.

Mercurius

A remedy for agitated states of mind. Hallucinations occur with impulses to run away and escape. There may be violent outbursts, and he is irritable and quick-tempered. All symptoms are worse at night, and from the heat of the bed. The breath is foul and offensive and he drips with sweat. A generalised tremor is present, often a chronic throat, ear, or skin infection which discharges pus.

Nux vomica

Delusional beliefs cause a great deal of anguish and are always worse in bed at night. There may be fantasies of violent destruction or murder. He is quick to anger and easily becomes violent, or a suicide attempt may be made, as rage is turned inwards. Sensitivity is marked, particularly to noise, bright lights, odour, touch and the presence of other people. There is an intense dislike of any form of restraint or contradiction.

Hypochondriacal and suspicious, levels of anxiety are high. There may be homicidal impulses. In most things, he tends to be hasty and precipitate, with sudden spasms of intense short-fuse anger, resentful and malicious. Muscular cramps, spasm, or areas of painful tension with chronic constipation are characteristic indications for prescribing this remedy.

Stramonium A remedy for acute, intense, delusional outbursts, the face red and swollen. The patient is excitable, often hypermanic, rushing about, laughing, tearful, shouting or singing. A high level of anxiety is often present, especially of being attacked. Speech is typically incoherent and muddled. Visual hallucinations, of dogs, small animals, insects, phantoms or ghosts, seem to surround or attack him, provoking feelings of terror. He is extremely fearful of being left alone. There is always an intense aversion to water or thinking about any form of liquid. All symptoms are worse at twilight.

157

Tarentula

For acute schizophrenic states, with restlessness, fear and agitation. A confused state of mind exists, marked by the most intense irritability. Moods shift quickly from anxiety and fear to destructive behaviour. Overall he is depressed, at times severely melancholic. The memory is weak. He tends to dislike bright colours and is irritated or fearful of red or green objects.

Veratrum alb

For severe delusional schizophrenic states, with confusion. The face is fearful, pale, drawn and cold. There are rapid mood changes, with an underlying sense of either hopeless despair, or delusions of grandeur (that he is Christ reincarnated). He is fearful of becoming blind, dumb, or dying from cancer. There may be violent outbursts and suicidal attempts. The patient always feels chilly and is covered in sweat. He may be exhausted to the point of collapse, at other times violent and excitable. Impulses to tear and destroy clothes or the sheets, may reach the point of frenzy.

SENILE CONFUSIONAL STATES

These are highly charged emotional states of the elderly, causing confusion, agitation, fear, delusional beliefs, mistrust, suspicion and often overactivity. A temporary change of personality may occur as a result of a severe infection, usually with a high temperature, or sometimes the result of a reaction to a prescribed medication. This is particularly likely to occur following a change of sedative, antibiotic, tranquilliser or anti-depressant, the adverse reaction affecting the mind and logical thinking processes. Other more serious causes are a brain tumour, or sometimes following an injury.

In others, confusion follows a change of environment, for example a move to a nursing home, or where illness necessitates a stay in hospital or any unfamiliar environment, where the change is misinterpreted. Relatives may be accused of trying to get them out of the home, gain access to savings, or sometimes it is interpreted as an attempt by neighbours to poison the food or air, or have them locked away. Loss of confidence is associated with fear and suspicion, and there may be attempts to run away from the ward or clinic. The whole situation is compounded where there is a communication problem, often related at this age to deafness, visual impairment, poor memory, and failure to comprehend what is happening and why a move is required.

For the elderly person, almost any change of environment is a stress and a trauma, leading to confusion and depersonalisation (loss of identity). To some extent this occurs with any adult, following a move to a new environment and it takes time to adjust psychologically, to 'find one's bearings'. With an elderly person, the adjustment may never occur.

Case report

An elderly lady in her 80's, lived in a granny flat attached to her son's house. She suddenly began accusing her daughter-in-law of taking cutlery from her kitchen, and deliberately moving or hiding her house linen. She became aggressive shouting at her in an accusing way, frightening the grandchildren, telling them their mother was a thief. In the past she had been quiet and affectionate, enjoying a good relationship with all members of the family including her daughter-in-law. There was no obvious cause for the mental condition, and she had not been on drugs, been ill or moved recently. The condition was clearly related to the sudden onset of senility. This led to confusion of mind, misrepresenting what was happening around her, and paranoid delusional ideas.

A similar confusional state may occur after the death of the spouse, sometimes with total denial of the event, or the need to be cared for in a residential home. It is common for senile patients to fabricate a situation in order to rationalise why the partner is no longer present. Another person, such as a nurse or care assistant, is often used to represent her, and called by her name. There is also a preoccupation with going home, endlessly repeating - 'You do know that I am going home tomorrow' although he is also aware that his house was sold to provide funds for sheltered accommodation or fees for the nursing home.

Sometimes old themes or disappointments from the past are raised, or the staff or family are addressed as a deceased brother or sister, who has not been talked about since childhood, but where there is still a nucleus of feelings and identity, and often a sense of loss and depression or anxiety.

The problem can be reduced or prevented, by giving plenty of warning before a major change is likely to happen, with frequent visits from the family, including the grandchildren. It is important to explain what is happening and why, trying to create a pleasant new environment, with a few favourite and familiar objects, perhaps a picture, cushions, a favourite chair or chest from home. If confusion is due to an infection, drug side-effect or sensitivity reaction, and hospitalisation is necessary, aim to get an elderly person back into their home and familiar environment as soon as possible. If a permanent stay is required, ensure that standards of care are professional and to a high level, with a minimum of isolation, and provision of maximum contact with other patients and staff, the environment sensitive and human. Contact with a friendly pet cat is often appreciated, and brings soothing relaxation and a sense of peace. Counselling and stimulation of creative interests are recommended and can be an important help to a confused mind. Always ensure a high level of nutrition, with regular vitamin and mineral supplements when indicated, particularly if underweight, when food is not absorbed well, or there is persistent diarrhoea or vomiting. Alcohol is usually best avoided, but when it has been part of a usual pattern, a little whisky in hot water at night often brings rest and helps sleep.

Character traits which aggravate the condition

There is a tendency towards narrow rigid attitudes, with failure to adapt and prepare for old age by developing new interests and outlets which fit in with any possible physical disabilities, for example deafness, poor vision, or arthritic problems. Isolation tends to worsen problems of confusion, usually because the memory is impaired. The situation is aggravated by mistrust and any tendency to avoid others.

Practical steps to improve things

Try to avoid isolating yourself, and not getting out to meet people. Aim to go to the local shops daily and try to make new friends. Join a local social club, and go along for the social contacts, someone to chat to for an hour or two, even if you are not a club person. If you are feeling down or anxious, always tell your family or helper, and ask to see your doctor.

Keep your intake of drugs minimal, and don't hoard drugs, or take them from time to time without first discussing it with your doctor. As soon as you feel better, stop taking any pills, unless these are strictly necessary for a heart, kidney, circulation, or other problem where regular drugs are needed, such as diabetes or thyroid problems. Try to keep contact with any friends you have known since childhood, even if you only write or see each other occasionally. Always talk about any odd beliefs or happenings you are experiencing, especially if you feel you are the victim of a plot. Aim to see your doctor regularly for a chat. Be open with him, and let him know how you are and discuss any worries with him. Don't stay cold, alone, and miserable, always ask for help. When you are feeling better, try to develop a new interest or hobby.

Remedies to consider:-

Anacardium

There are variable moods, at times cheerful, then depressed, irritable, or melancholic. Other feelings are of isolation, indifference, lack of confidence, paranoid anxieties with suspicion. The memory is extremely poor, often unable to recall names or words.

Argentum nit

A remedy for confusional states of the elderly with phobic anxiety features. There is total intolerance of all forms of heat.

Baryta carb

This is useful for pre-senile states of dementia, with infantile behaviour patterns. He is tired, fearful of strangers, new situations, often pessimistic. Memory is poor.

Lycopodium

Indicated for distracted states, and a 'butterfly' mind, darting from one subject to another, and leading to confusion. He may spend hours gazing out of the window, looking at nothing, lost in thought. Anguish in the pit of the stomach, and depression are usually worse from 4.00-8.00pm. He tends to be clumsy and accident-prone.

Natrum mur

For weeping, depressed, irritable moods of the elderly. He dreads all forms of intellectual work and is unable to concentrate. The mind is confused. Dull mentally, memory is poor for recent events.

Nux vomica

For silent, tense, irritable and confused states of mind. At times impatient and violent, he is oversensitive to noise, odours and bright light. Hypochondriacal, he is full of complaints, miserable and pessimistic, with no patience for work. Concentration is also difficult and he misuses words. Problems of constipation may become linked to delusional fears of becoming totally blocked.

Sulphur

Indicated when there is a mixture of confusion and agitation, taken up with old and past resentments. He is often untidy and dirty, because of self-neglect, at the same time idealising old clothes or rags as beautiful. The memory is weak, especially for names and places. Much of the time, he is depressed and tearful, rambling in a vague, speculative, fanciful way about meaningless ideas. At other times he is arrogant and full of his own importance.

SHORT FUSE IRRITABILITY

This is not strictly a psychological illness, but it usually reflects frustration due to severe underlying pressure and tension. It is often the build-up of unexpressed emotion which leads to tension states or depressive illness. Irritability and poor control of emotions become associated with feelings of futility and failure. There is often a high degree of intolerance, or petty criticism of the family. Bullying, insults and abuse are felt to be more effective in controlling others than discussion and dialogue. Much of this is the result of underlying rigid attitudes, insecurity, stubborn pride, and lack of confidence, although this is rarely admitted to.

There is a tendency to set impossibly high standards of achievement for self and others, which inevitably causes disappointment, with a tendency to blame others. There may be a 'slave driver' mentality towards work, deadlines, and cleanliness, intolerant of disorder or mess. The emphasis is on appearance, neatness, results, rather than a change in attitudes and a gentler more creative tolerant approach to life. If you do have a tendency towards rigid unreasonable attitudes, with obsessional controls, it adds to the pressures you place upon yourself, as well as others.

At times, the whole world can seem to revolve around caution and order, not taking risks, keeping everything the same. There may be dislike of spending money and anything new is seen as a threat or extravagance. This may include money spent on furniture, a holiday or travelling, driving lessons, or on the car.
There may be similar attitudes to buying clothes, or anything new for the home. Each new purchase is felt

to be a threat, greeted with ' Why do you want that ? You don't need it, it is a waste of money'. There is often an underlying fear of the partner becoming more independent, and the changes and demands this may bring.

Beneath the reactions of irritability and temper, there are usually feelings of fear and anxiety, trapped by a social or financial situation, or that any change or decision will be for the worse. When irritability becomes a problem, most of the day may be spent preoccupied with the limitations of others, making life a misery for them, rather than admitting your own fears and indecision. Alcohol considerably increases any angry outbursts, because it intensifies feelings of depression and frustration.

Accident proneness often presents as a recurrent low-back problem, frozen shoulder or tendon injury. These are often due to the extremes of tension and rigidity which accompany even the simplest movement. Exhaustion or sexual difficulties, such as premature ejaculation, failure to achieve an orgasm, or impotence, are other common problems because physically as well as psychologically, every aspect of life is pressurised.

Character traits which aggravate the condition

There is a tendency to be wooden and rigid in all aspects of self-expression and spontaneity. The basic problem is often one of excessive self-control, and feeling vulnerable. There is nearly always scope for greater flexibility and a more creative life-style.

Practical steps to improve things

Aim to be easy and relaxed in everything you do, less demanding and intense in your expectations and relationships, including those outside your job and immediate family. Try to be less of a perfectionist in attitudes towards yourself, less dramatic and disappointed, when everything does not go according to (your) plan. Don't expect so much from others. Relax more and take time off for enjoyable leisure pursuits such as walking, cycling, swimming and other sports.

If you feel irritable, about to explode, unable to control your feelings, try to see how this fits into an overall pattern, finding others incompetent and a failure, rather than admitting your own feelings of failure and frustration. Try walking away from situations where you are becoming over-heated and losing control. This may help you find a better perspective and more insight, without giving in to another explosive outburst. These are unhelpful psychologically, because they reinforce the pattern, and physically, by increasing blood-pressure, they may put your overall health at risk. Also it does not help you look at the underlying causes of the problem and how to understand and solve it. Try to remember that each outburst is ultimately a weakness, related to poor controls, and harms you psychologically. Consider regular meditation and massage to help you relax more.

167

Remedies to consider:-

Causticum Extremely sympathetic, with a tendency to nervous irritability. Angry and over-reacting to a minor event, the moods vary from depression to peevish fretfulness. Restless feelings are usually worse in the morning.

Chamomilla There are irritable moods with whining, excitable, restlessness. Constantly complaining and moaning if he does not have his own way. All symptoms are worse from heat and at night.

Graphites For tearful, depressed mood-swings. The typical morning irritability is aggravated by the least thing.

Lilium tig Tearful, depressive moods occur, with irritability and impulses to strike out or to hit others who annoy. He is often anxious and tense on waking.

Nux vomica There is short-fuse irritability with over-zealous attitudes. Indigestion, nausea and chronic constipation are other common problems.

Staphisagria A remedy for extreme irritation.

168

SUICIDAL THOUGHTS AND IMPULSES

These are common at moments of extreme stress, usually associated with feelings of rage, frustration, depression, or sometimes as part of an acute grief reaction. Often there has been a major disappointment which cannot be adequately expressed, or there is an overwhelming impulse to hit out in destructive anger, sometimes at others, but often at the self. Anger may have been felt for years, but never expressed, or it may have never been easy to come to terms with or show certain feelings, particularly rage, frustration, disapproval or jealousy. As a child, these feelings may have been strong and an appropriate reaction to provocation at the time, but at the same time taboo, because they were too intense, uncontrollable or destructive. Feelings of rage may have been turned inwards and never shown. Adult or adolescent suicidal impulses may be a continuation of a childhood pattern, and self-destructive tendencies. Frequently the parents were intolerant of any outward show of aggression, either because they had poor controls themselves, or they did not know how to handle anger and repressed it in themselves and in their children. In some instances, one of the parents was depressed during childhood and took an overdose, or threatened to, when under pressure or not in control. This form of behaviour is essentially a manipulation and may have occurred during early childhood only to be repeated in later life.

Just as anger may have been suppressed over the years, so too, feelings of love, need and affection may also have been denied (or internalised), including the need to cry or to grieve.

Suicidal preoccupations, or an actual attempt, may be a call for help, a signal of need for closeness, greater understanding and support, as well as a gesture of rage and frustration. Any threat of suicide should be taken seriously, whatever the age of the person, as tragedies occur, even in childhood, and the most staged gesture can go wrong and end in disaster. For this reason every family should see a threat or talk of suicide as a signal for much more individual talking time, until they are quite certain that an improvement in confidence and mood has occurred. If a suicidal threat is part of a psychotic illness, for example a manic-depressive illness, or when a diagnosis of schizophrenia has been made, then the family should discuss this with the doctor or therapist who is in charge of treatment.

An increase in melancholic thoughts and suicidal impulses may be related to the side-effect of a prescribed drug, and this is a further reason to ensure that the doctor involved in the treatment knows about such threats, and has the time to make any adjustment required to the medication he has given. Such risks do not occur however with homoeopathic treatments, and are only a complication of certain conventional drugs.

Character traits which aggravate the condition

There is a tendency to internalise (deny) any powerful feelings and reactions, particularly those relating to hurt, disappointment, need, and frustration. Anger or tantrums during childhood may not have been tolerated by the parents or allowed any outward form of expression. At times, unbearable tension, rage and anguish may be felt as a desire to hit out, feeling like a volcano about to explode.

Practical steps to improve things

Try to express your feelings directly, and as they occur, not after the event, or becoming angry with yourself because of what you wanted to say, but didn't. Biting your lip may be diplomatic, but it is not recommended for psychological health. Aim to express all your emotions at the time, especially frustration, rage, grief, disappointment, and try to put these into better perspective, including any self-destructive impulses. Talk more openly with your partner, friends and family when you feel depressed and try to detect the anger behind a suicidal thought or impulse. Always clarify what you are avoiding by directing aggression at yourself, rather than using it positively. See suicidal thoughts as a move to avoid or annihilate a particular problem area, which may be painful and inconvenient, but nevertheless needs resolving. Consider it also as a flight from the challenge of change, new directions and personal growth, the need to make a fundamental shift in your life-style.

Remedies to consider:-

Aurum met

Irritable, depressed, despondent, with compulsive thoughts of suicide. A sense of anguish occurs in the chest, also palpitations and rheumatic joint pains.

Natrum mur

A remedy for extremes of anguish and despair. A profound state of depression is accompanied by exhaustion. The mood is aggravated by social contact, sympathy or consolation.

Nux vomica

Irritability with depression, and impulses to violence or self-destruction. Everything is conceived in extremes, and self-control is usually unreliable.

Platina

For an arrogant, superior state of mind, at times depressed and weeping. Impulses to violence or self-destruction are worse in the evening, improved by exercise and fresh air.

Pulsatilla

There is a changeable, very unpredictable state of mind, varying from extremes of anguish and sadness, to laughter or anger. An overdose may be used as a gesture to try to attract attention.

TENSION STATES

Whenever tension builds up and is not allowed an external expression through dialogue or action, it may cause symptoms of varying degrees of discomfort and severity. When the build-up is acute, it can lead to a nervous breakdown or a severe psychological illness. The tense person often feels in an extreme state of unrest and pain, both physical and mental, making relaxation or concentration difficult, if not impossible.

There is usually a clear cause for the tension, resulting in a profound sense of oppression. This interferes with all the normal physiological functioning, causing the bowels to be loose, urination frequent, digestion upset, stomach cramps, windy indigestion, pain after eating, nausea and sometimes lack of appetite. Sleep is interfered with, not getting off to sleep for hours, or sometimes waking in the early hours, with a sense of apprehension and anguish, eventually dropping off again about 4-5.00 am. and feeling exhausted. The tension may involve the heart, causing palpitations (awareness of the heart beating), missed or irregular beats, at times needle-like, pricking chest pains which come and go and a sensation of weakness or collapse. Weight loss may occur, as there is little or no interest in food. The general state of health is run down because of failure to eat nourishing meals. Energy and reserves are further drained by failure to relax. Persistent low backache is a common symptom of tension, which may become incapacitating, causing months of pain and misery, often worse for any treatment given. Localised muscle pains, aching discomfort, spasms or cramp, a frozen shoulder, recurrent lumbago, neck stiffness, are other common manifestations of this condition.

The cause of the tension is not always clear. For some, there has been a recent change of lifestyle, due to early retirement, being made redundant, a business failure, a move to a less healthy environment, or feeling insecure and depressed after the loss or illness of a partner. Other common factors are divorce and the breakdown of a relationship. All of these may cause tension, anxiety and fear, with feelings of vulnerability. In the past, there may have been an over-dependant relationship, all initiative and decision-making left to the partner. When more responsibility has to be taken after loss or separation from the partner, this can lead to feelings of insecurity and fear, leading to agitation and unbearable tension.

Stiff and rigid, restless pacing, up and down, like a tiger in a cage, may be the only way to find some relief from the tension. The problem may be compounded by a hypochondriacal conviction that there is an underlying physical illness, trying many different treatments, all of which end in failure or worsen the condition. There may be a deeply held conviction that the condition will get worse, especially if the cause or diagnosis has not been clearly explained to the patient who, fearing the worst, is convinced he is dying.

Character traits which aggravate the condition

There is a tendency to keep feelings inside, reluctant to talk in sufficient depth about emotions, anxieties and doubts as they occur and when they should be shared. Rigid attitudes lead to an accumulation of tension, which builds up because of failure to relax or let go. The overall approach to life may be obsessional, too orderly, priority only given to neatness and control, rather than relaxation and open sharing. Everything is predictable and shipshape, at a time when emotionally the reverse is true. Feelings of anger, loss, grief, frustration, and resentment, are not given full expression, in case they become overwhelming, or make you look weak or foolish. Pride is also an underlying factor which underpins tension, causing inflexibility, and making a positive healthy adjustment more difficult.

Practical steps to improve things

Try to share more and be more open. Practise letting go of feelings and problems as they occur, with your partner, friends, and the family. At the same time, don't be over-dramatic, to avoid swamping or overloading your partner with excessive feelings he has to back away from, in order to survive. This does not mean repressing or controlling emotions or lack of spontaneity, but some consideration and caring, as you share and give out more of yourself. If you are worried and can't immediately resolve a problem, try distancing yourself from it for a day or so, but always keeping problems in perspective. Try to see how you limit yourself, and find ways of avoiding repetitive patterns which in the past have led to a build-up of tension. Look for areas of change and development where you can feel more fulfilled, relaxed and at peace.

Remedies to consider:-

Aconitum A remedy for sudden acute states of tension, associated with fear, anxiety, restless agitation, and nervous irritability. The face is hot and bright red. There is intolerance of touch or palpation.

Arsenicum For tension states with anxiety. The person is always chilly, craving heat, the face pale, thin and drawn. Fussy and restless because of tension, he often feels weak and exhausted. Burning pains are characteristic, occurring anywhere in the body. Fears of going out or being alone, are always worse for consolation.

Lycopodium Indicated for anticipatory fears. The forehead is lined and wrinkled from chronic anxiety and frowning. There is a constant state of anguish and tension. He often prefers to be in his room, but dreads being alone in the house. Most symptoms are worse from 4-8.00 pm. He craves sweet foods, especially chocolate, as a comfort from anxiety and the uncertainty of life.

Natrum mur   Indicated for chronic tension states, usually associated with a weeping depression. He is thin, always chilly, often feeling worse from heat. Moods are constantly changeable, and he is never fully confident or at ease in a social situation, wanting sympathy, but is worse for consolation or close contact. He tends to be rather indifferent, a loner, and over-sensitive, without much sense of humour.

Nux vomica   A remedy where the underlying personality is over-intense and anxious. He easily becomes resentful and irritable, having a short-fuse temper, at the same time malicious. Because of chronic digestive problems, the face and nose are frequently bright red. He is usually constipated. In addition, there is hypersensitivity to touch, noise, bright lights and odours. All symptoms are worse in the early night hours, usually at 3.00 am.

TOXIC STATES

These may occur because of poisoning, involving the brain or nervous system, for example, the result of bacterial food poisoning or a very high temperature during an acute infection, such as meningitis or influenza. But there is also a risk from a sensitivity or allergic reaction to certain prescribed drugs. Excesses of some of the common social props, especially alcohol, but also illicit drugs such as opium, L.S.D., 'speed', Ecstasy, and adolescent glue-sniffing, may lead to a confused toxic state of mind which may be fatal. It is normal when recovering from an anaesthetic, before the body is able to excrete the anaesthetic from the system and much worse when the patient is elderly or allergic to the drugs used.

Toxic fungi, mistakenly taken to be edible, will similarly cause an acute toxic state of mind, sometimes a brief delusional illness, with restlessness or even violence. A similar illness may occur when poisonous plants or berries are taken, either as play 'sweets' by children, or used to make a 'herbal tea' by adults, who mistakenly believe they have health-giving properties.

In most cases, a toxic state of confusion ceases as soon as the drug is withdrawn, or there is recovery from whatever is causing the toxic state. The condition can be easily differentiated from a schizophrenic or manic-depressive illness, because of the hot flushed skin, high temperature and often fixed dilated pupils.

Toxic states are a common problem of the elderly, especially following a high, or sometimes normal adult dosage, of certain prescribed drugs, particularly sedatives, anti-histamines, anti-depressants, sometimes antibiotics or pain killers. Certain drugs tend to accumulate quickly within the body tissues to toxic levels, because of sluggish kidney and liver action, often the result of age, previous damage, surgery or infection. This slows the normal breakdown, detoxifying and elimination action of these organs, which protects the brain and nervous system from becoming poisoned. The condition may become chronic, the toxic state persisting in a mild or intermittent form for months after the drug has been eliminated from the system. In most cases there is a full recovery, but symptoms may last for months or years after stopping a drug, the body not feeling 'right' and the general health may become permanently impaired.

Case report
Two years after stopping a particular anti-depressant, a young woman in her 20's, still felt unwell, unable to work or make plans, in a drugged sedated state, constantly exhausted, with blurred vision, both pupils dilated. Her mouth felt constantly dry, the tongue white and coated. Most of the time, her stomach was bloated and she developed persistent constipation. The colour of her skin had also changed and become yellow, although before taking the drug, it had been a healthy clear pink. She felt cold, her muscles ached and she was unable to cry or properly express feelings, as if all her emotions were dulled and her whole physiology had changed. With homoeopathic treatment, there was a marked improvement in levels of anxiety and fear, with increased energy and concentration.

Character traits which aggravate the condition

An immature tendency to idealise and be over-trusting of authority figures, naively believing, that whatever is recommended must be right. There is weakness of self-trust and self-knowledge, also intuitive skills, knowing what suits you best as an individual, your constitutional make-up, and what is harmful. This makes you vulnerable to exploitation at many levels, and puts you more at risk.

Practical steps to improve things

Try to value yourself more, to know yourself better, and not taking everything to the letter or to extremes. In this way you will feel less anxious and vulnerable when under pressure. Your individuality matters at all levels, and you need to find out what works best for your particular constitution. What may have been tolerated in the past, may not be right for you now, particularly as you become more mature. If you feel unwell after taking a particular drug, always discuss this with your doctor, and don't persist with it for weeks or months, especially if you feel confused or exhausted. Avoid any remedy or therapy that is not helping you to heal, develop, grow and expand physically and psychologically. This includes food, alcohol, and prescribed medicines. Become more questioning and discerning. Don't just accept or take something as right for you, because the man who prescribes it wears a white coat or a suit. Try to develop more discerning skills and rely on your intuition. Find a simple, natural approach to life which does not put you at risk.

Remedies to consider:-

Aconitum   Useful for acute states of shock, associated with overwhelming fear.

Arnica   Indicated for restless states of shock, constantly twisting and turning, complaining the bed is too hard. Physically he feels bruised, usually in the right side of the chest. He is also hurt and bruised psychologically.

Arsenicum   A remedy for states of exhaustion, the patient pale, ice cold and craving heat. He is restless and agitated and full of fears. There is an irritable bowel problem, with diarrhoea and burning pains throughout the body.

Nux vomica   Indicated when there is a combination of irritability, with spasms of colicky pain and constipation.

Opium   He is apprehensive and sleepy, to the point of becoming sluggish or falling into a coma. The face is bright red, the eyes staring. He complains of severe temporal headache. There are problems of very obstinate constipation.

Phosphorus   This remedy is helpful when the patient has liver damage. He is chilly and pale, the skin yellow or jaundiced, the stools chalky white in colour. There is a tendency to bleed easily. Ice-cold drinks are craved.

Pyrogen   There is a high temperature. The pulse slows as the fever rises, but becomes more rapid if there is only a moderate rise in temperature. There is an agitated mental state, with apprehension, over-talkative, irritable, or delirious. The breath is fetid, the head covered in sweat.

Sulphur   A remedy for chronic toxic states, the appearance neglected and untidy, the face red, skin infected. There is an offensive chronic diarrhoea. The mind tends to ramble, with vague, disjointed, speculative ideas. All symptoms are worse from heat, eating, washing and sleeping.

The specific drug which initially caused the toxic state, taken as a homoeopathic potency.

VIOLENCE

This is a common symptom of psychological illness, directed either at the self or others. Violence is often the result of a build-up of tension which cannot be released other than by an uncontrollable physical, sometimes psychological, act of violence. It may occur during any acute emotional situation, where there is a lack of meaningful dialogue, misunderstanding and intense pent-up feelings.

Violence tends to occur when under pressure, especially during a divorce, concerns about job security, redundancy, or any form of financial anxiety or hardship. It frequently reflects a lack of confidence, unable to express ideas or emotions adequately, and lacking the assertive skills to express them. This may contribute to an uncontrollable build-up of:- frustration, anger, impatience, impotence and rage, which then acts as a trigger to violence.

The problem may have occurred over many years, starting with temper tantrums as a child, which at the times, were not checked or disciplined in a firm non-violent way. If these 'paid off' psychologically, successfully manipulating the mother, (the child getting his own way), then violence may have continued into adolescence as sulky outbursts, truancy, delinquency and bullying. Often the violent adult was bullied or abused as a child, the adult simply repeating what was handed out to him whenever he was in the way or made himself heard.

The problem may have first occurred after a severe accident, causing psychological or physical damage, for example, a head injury with concussion. But any major injury, particularly one involving loss of limb, can lead to a change of personality and violence. Other major contributing factors are:- pre-senile changes, sometimes occurring at an early age (from the mid-fifties onwards), jealousy, suspicion, lack of trust, pollution, sustained or intermittent noise, and overcrowding.

Extreme or rigid attitudes, tend to underpin violence, and these are often a key issue in any form of mental illness. Violent outbursts sometimes occur during psychiatric treatment, as the patient regresses, or attempts are made to explore the underlying causes and motivations behind his illness.

A common factor in violence is the need to find a scapegoat for feelings of inadequacy or failure. Many focus the cause of their limitations upon others, failing to see that the fault lies in their own personal attitudes which act as a brake on life. Rigid intolerant attitudes of resentment and jealousy, bullying or abuse, may develop towards a half-brother or sister. A live-in partner's child is especially at risk. Violence is particularly common in any institution, such as prison, hostel, community home or boarding school, where there is a lack of privacy, with overcrowding, the absence of parental restraints or demonstrable love and affection.

Alcohol and drug abuse, are the commonest causes of violence in the home, associated with underlying feelings of depression, frustration, failure or inadequacy, which exacerbates the violent behaviour.

There may be a suicidal attempt, sometimes as a result of the side-effects of a particular prescribed drug, or because of a delusional state of mind. This may be due to drug abuse, particularly after taking L.S.D. or 'speed'. The risks are increased when drugs are mixed with alcohol.

Violence at the wheel is increasingly becoming a problem area. It constitutes a form of social violence, with risk taking, speeding, cutting-in and shouting abuse. Sometimes actual fights, physical threats or violence towards other road users may occur. In the US recently, shoot-outs and gun attacks at the wheel, have occurred in several cities, injuring or killing motorists.

Case report
A young family drove home recently from the surgery after a consultation. The husband passed another car. Without provocation, the other driver became incensed and followed them for miles. When they pulled into a garage for petrol, he pulled in beside them, and in front of the wife and young children, pulled out a knife, and gashed the paint-work along the side of the car.

Violence towards the self, and suicide attempts are other expressions of impatience, frustration and tension. It is not uncommon for a psychologically ill patient to cut his arms or wrists and to violently rub or pick at his nails and skin, causing damage. The most common causes for this kind of behaviour are feelings of anger,

185

isolation, confusion, and despair. A severe mourning reaction after the death of a partner may sometimes lead to violence and suicide. Fear of aging and dependency, associated with stubborn pride, can also end in violence. A suicide pact, to be implemented at a certain age, may have been planned years before, to avoid aging and dependency, and is a form of delayed violence. Anger at a difficult or seemingly unjust situation in the home may also lead to violent arguments, rage and frustration, especially if discussion is limited or impossible.

Often the individual involved has never felt able to cope verbally with disagreements, or any challenge to his authority. Violence seems to be the only way to find immediate relief from unbearable internal tension, or to control an impossible family or work situation.

Other reasons for violence are of a more delusional nature, due to psychotic thinking, during an acute mental illness. Threats of violence, may sometimes involve the elderly. They are usually directed towards the self, as a suicidal attempt. More rarely a tragedy occurs involving a neighbour or a close member of the family, the aggression and violence due to a senile confusional state.

Character traits which aggravate the condition

Impatience, lack of tolerance and weakness in self-confidence. A tendency to hit-out first and talk afterwards. Problems of violence indicate a high-risk, rigid approach to life and are usually based on fear and lack of trust.

Practical steps to improve things

Practise staying calm in all situations, especially if you feel provoked or are losing control. Talk every emotional situation through and express yourself clearly. Walk away from provocative situations and try to relax if you start to feel tense or anxious. Regular, (at least three times a week) periods of meditation are recommended, and apply this when under pressure. Avoid being a workaholic, working late, getting overtired, bringing work home at weekends or on holiday. Alcohol is best avoided completely, if you cannot drink in moderation, or it provokes a violent reaction. If you are feeling worried, then talk about it before it becomes a problem. Don't allow feelings to build-up into major areas of tension and resentment. If you want to build a less violent society, treat all children, including your step-children, with respect and consideration and don't humiliate or beat them. You can punish a child fairly and in a manner he will accept and understand without threats or smacking. Asking the child to go to his room or to stay seated is often sufficient for simple misdemeanours. Cutting down on pocket money or an outing are other ways of showing disapproval without resorting to violence. Every child learns and identifies with the emotional reactions of his parents, with what is done, rather than said. Violence to a child, can set the pattern for adult aggression and abuse, sometimes causing damage for generations.

Remedies to consider:-

Aurum met   There is anguish and short-fuse violent rage or anger. At other times there may be a severe depression with suicidal impulses.

Hyoscyamus   For excitable, restless states with confusion, jealousy or suspicion. Violence may occur, and a tendency to bite.

Nux vomica   Short-fuse irritability occurs, with poor controls and impulses to violence. Beneath the aggression, lies a problem of depression and often deep-seated frustrations.

Sepia   There is extreme fatigue, indifference to loved ones and a profound depression with impulses to strike-out. Irritability is increased by thunder, consolation, or physical contact.

Stramonium   Rapidly changing, noisy, confused, excitable moods occur. There is a dislike of bright lights and water.

Tarentula   For tearful, hysterical agitation and depressive mood swings. Restless, aggressive behaviour leads to violence.

INDEX

HOMOEOPATHY

Understanding Homoeopathy

The revised second edition of this comprehensive book explains in clear, simple terms the basic principles of homoeopathy, which can be readily understood by the beginner. The author outlines the approach, indications, and choice of remedies for the common health problems of the family.

Talking About Homoeopathy

An invaluable reference book for anyone wishing to understand homoeopathy. The book covers a variety of topics of general interest which offer a deeper understanding and a more challenging awareness of homoeopathy, its indications, potential and scope of action.

The Principles, Art and Practice of Homoeopathy

A book which explains in simple language the principles of homoeopathic practice and prescribing. It includes chapters on :- Dosage, Potency, First and Second Prescriptions, Homoeopathic History Taking and The Consultation. A second section is concerned with Constitutional Prescribing, and the role of homoeopathy in the treatment of Cancer.

PSYCHOLOGY

Emotional Health

A unique and major study of the most common emotional problems facing society in the twentieth century. It identifies their causes and symptoms, and then explains the best, practical, self-help steps that can be taken to solve them. Simple guidelines are given in order to promote healthier attitudes, changes in specific problem areas, and better psychological perspectives.

Personal Growth and Creativity

A guide to the most effective ways to stimulate and develop personal creativity in order to bring about positive change in creative outlook. The book offers practical guidelines that will lead to constructive results.

RISKS OF MODERN LIVING

The Side-Effects Book

This books describes in detail the most common hazards of our pressurised society, the props used and their risk to health. Chapters include: Developmental Stages of life, Stress and the Home, Sexuality, Over-The-Counter Drugs, Health Products and Vitamins, Medically Prescribed Drugs, Surgical and Cosmetic Procedures, Immunisation, Food and Diet, Social Addictions, Holidays and the Sun, Travel, Sport, Occupations, Animals and Plants, Household Products, Pesticides, Drugs of Dependence and Misuse, Pollution.

Please send s.a.e. for a list of other titles available.